DATE DUE

Does Stress Cause Psychiatric Illness?

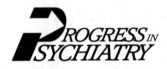

PROGRESS *IN* **PSYCHIATRY**

Number 46

David Spiegel, M.D.
Series Editor

Does Stress Cause Psychiatric Illness?

Edited by
Carolyn M. Mazure, Ph.D.

Washington, DC
London, England

Manufactured in the United States of America on acid-free paper

First Edition   98 97 96 95   4 3 2 1

American Psychiatric Press, Inc.
1400 K Street, N.W., Washington, DC   20005

Library of Congress Cataloging-in-Publication Data
Does stress cause psychiatric illness? / edited by Carolyn M. Mazure.
     p. cm. — (Progress in psychiatry series ; #46)
   Includes bibliographical references and index.
   ISBN 0-88048-482-9 (alk. paper)
   1. Mental illness—Etiology. 2. Stress (Psychology) I. Mazure,
Carolyn M. II. Series.
   [DNLM: 1. Stress, Psychological. 2. Mental Disorders—etiology.
W1 PR6781L no. 46 1995 / WM 172 D653 1995]
RC455.4.S87D64 1995
616.89′071—dc20
DNLM/DLC
for Library of Congress   94-22178
                                                                          CIP

British Library Cataloguing in Publication Data
A CIP record is available from the British Library.

Contents

Contributors

Alan Breier, M.D.
Chief, Unit of Pathophysiology and Treatment, Experimental Therapeutics Branch, National Institute of Mental Health, Bethesda, Maryland

J. Douglas Bremner, M.D.
Assistant Professor, Department of Psychiatry, Yale University School of Medicine; and Research Psychiatrist, West Haven Veterans Administration Medical Center, West Haven, Connecticut

Dennis S. Charney, M.D.
Professor and Associate Chair for Research, Department of Psychiatry, Yale University School of Medicine; and Director, Division of Clinical Neurosciences, National Center for Posttraumatic Stress Disorder, West Haven Veterans Administration Medical Center, West Haven, Connecticut

Bonnie S. Dansky, Ph.D.
Assistant Professor, Department of Psychiatry and Behavioral Sciences, National Crime Victims Research and Treatment Center, Medical University of South Carolina, Charleston, South Carolina

Bruce P. Dohrenwend, Ph.D.
Professor, Department of Psychiatry and School of Public Health, Columbia University; and Chief, Department of Social Psychiatry, New York State Psychiatric Institute, New York, New York

Benjamin G. Druss, M.D.
Mental Health Services Research Fellow, Departments of Psychiatry and Public Health, Yale University School of Medicine, New Haven, Connecticut

Sherry A. Falsetti, Ph.D.
Instructor, Department of Psychiatry and Behavioral
Sciences, National Crime Victims Research and Treatment
Center, Clinical Research Section, Medical University of
South Carolina, Charleston, South Carolina

Constance L. Hammen, Ph.D.
Professor of Psychology and Psychiatry and Biobehavioral
Sciences, University of California, Los Angeles,
Los Angeles, California

Selby Jacobs, M.D., M.P.H.
Professor, Department of Psychiatry, Yale University
School of Medicine, New Haven, Connecticut

Dean G. Kilpatrick, Ph.D.
Professor, Department of Psychiatry and Behavioral
Sciences; Director, National Crime Victims Research and
Treatment Center; Director, Psychology Internship
Program, Medical University of South Carolina, Charleston,
South Carolina

Kathleen Kim, M.D., M.P.H.
Assistant Professor, Department of Psychiatry, Yale
University School of Medicine, New Haven, Connecticut

Marsha L. Kline, Ph.D.
Associate Research Scientist, Department of Psychiatry,
Yale University School of Medicine, New Haven,
Connecticut

David J. Kupfer, M.D.
Professor and Chairman, Department of Psychiatry,
Western Psychiatric Institute and Clinic, University of
Pittsburgh School of Medicine, Pittsburgh, Pennsylvania

Bruce G. Link, Ph.D.
Associate Professor, School of Public Health, Columbia
University, New York, New York

R. Bruce Lydiard, M.D., Ph.D.
Professor, Department of Psychiatry and Behavioral
Sciences; Medical Director, Clinical Research Section and
Anxiety Disorders Program; Co-Director, Psychiatry
Pharmacology Program, Medical University of South
Carolina, Charleston, South Carolina

Carolyn M. Mazure, Ph.D.
Associate Professor, Department of Psychiatry, Yale
University School of Medicine, New Haven, Connecticut

Heidi S. Resnick, Ph.D.
Associate Professor, Department of Psychiatry and
Behavioral Sciences, National Crime Victims Research and
Treatment Center, Medical University of South Carolina,
Charleston, South Carolina

Patrick E. Shrout, Ph.D.
Professor, Department of Psychology, New York
University, New York, New York

Andrew E. Skodol, M.D.
Associate Professor of Clinical Psychiatry, Department of
Psychiatry, Columbia University; and Psychiatrist III, New
York State Psychiatric Institute, New York, New York

David L. Snow, Ph.D.
Associate Professor of Psychology, Department of
Psychiatry and the Child Study Center, Yale University
School of Medicine, New Haven, Connecticut

Steven M. Southwick, M.D.
Associate Professor, Department of Psychiatry, Yale
University School of Medicine; and Director, Posttraumatic
Stress Disorder Program, West Haven Veterans
Administration Medical Center, West Haven, Connecticut

Ann Stueve, Ph.D.
Assistant Professor, School of Public Health, Columbia
University, New York, New York

Introduction to the Progress in Psychiatry Series

The Progress in Psychiatry Series is designed to capture in print the excitement that comes from assembling a diverse group of experts from various locations to examine in detail the newest information about a developing aspect of psychiatry. This series emerged as a collaboration between the American Psychiatric Association's (APA) Scientific Program Committee and the American Psychiatric Press, Inc. Great interest is generated by a number of the symposia presented each year at the APA annual meeting, and we realized that much of the information presented there, carefully assembled by people who are deeply immersed in a given area, would unfortunately not appear together in print. The symposia sessions at the annual meetings provide an unusual opportunity for experts who otherwise might not meet on the same platform to share their diverse viewpoints for a period of 3 hours. Some new themes are repeatedly reinforced and gain credence, whereas in other instances disagreements emerge, enabling the audience and now the reader to reach informed decisions about new directions in the field. The Progress in Psychiatry Series allows us to publish and capture some of the best of the symposia and thus provide an in-depth treatment of specific areas that might not otherwise be presented in broader review formats.

Psychiatry is, by nature, an interface discipline, combining the study of mind and brain, of individual and social environments, of the humane and the scientific. Therefore, progress in the field is rarely linear—it often comes from unexpected sources. Furthermore, new developments emerge from an array of viewpoints that do not necessarily provide immediate agreement but rather expert examination of the issues. We intend to present innovative ideas and data that will enable you, the reader, to participate in this process.

We believe the Progress in Psychiatry Series will provide you with an opportunity to review timely, new information in specific fields of interest as they are developing. We hope you find that the excitement of the presentations is captured in the written word and that this book proves to be informative and enjoyable reading.

David Spiegel, M.D.
Series Editor
Progress in Psychiatry Series

Progress in Psychiatry Series Titles

Does Stress Cause Psychiatric Illness? (#46)
Edited by Carolyn M. Mazure, Ph.D.

Biological and Neurobehavioral Studies of Borderline Personality Disorder (#45)
Edited by Kenneth R. Silk, M.D.

Severe Depressive Disorders (#44)
Edited by Leon Grunhaus, M.D., and John F. Greden, M.D.

Clinical Advances in Monoamine Oxidase Inhibitor Therapies (#43)
Edited by Sidney H. Kennedy, M.D., F.R.C.P.C.

Catecholamine Function in Posttraumatic Stress Disorder: Emerging Concepts (#42)
Edited by M. Michele Murburg, M.D.

Management and Treatment of Insanity Acquittees: A Model for the 1990s (#41)
Edited by Joseph D. Bloom, M.D., and Mary H. Williams, M.S., J.D.

Chronic Fatigue and Related Immune Deficiency Syndromes (#40)
Edited by Paul J. Goodnick, M.D., and Nancy G. Klimas, M.D.

Psychopharmacology and Psychobiology of Ethnicity (#39)
Edited by Keh-Ming Lin, M.D., M.P.H., Russell E. Poland, Ph.D., and Gayle Nakasaki, M.S.W.

Electroconvulsive Therapy: From Research to Clinical Practice (#38)
Edited by C. Edward Coffey, M.D.

Treatment Strategies for Refractory Depression (#25)
Edited by Steven P. Roose, M.D., and
Alexander H. Glassman, M.D.

Biological Rhythms, Mood Disorders, Light Therapy, and the Pineal Gland (#24)
Edited by Mohammad Shafii, M.D., and
Sharon Lee Shafii, R.N., B.S.N.

Family Environment and Borderline Personality Disorder (#23)
Edited by Paul Skevington Links, M.D.

Amino Acids in Psychiatric Disease (#22)
Edited by Mary Ann Richardson, Ph.D.

Serotonin in Major Psychiatric Disorders (#21)
Edited by Emil F. Coccaro, M.D., and Dennis L. Murphy, M.D.

Personality Disorders: New Perspectives on Diagnostic Validity (#20)
Edited by John M. Oldham, M.D.

Biological Assessment and Treatment of Posttraumatic Stress Disorder (#19)
Edited by Earl L. Giller, Jr., M.D., Ph.D.

Depression in Schizophrenia (#18)
Edited by Lynn E. DeLisi, M.D.

Depression and Families: Impact and Treatment (#17)
Edited by Gabor I. Keitner, M.D.

Depressive Disorders and Immunity (#16)
Edited by Andrew H. Miller, M.D.

Treatment of Tricyclic-Resistant Depression (#15)
Edited by Irl L. Extein, M.D.

Current Approaches to the Prediction of Violence (#14)
Edited by David A. Brizer, M.D., and Martha L. Crowner, M.D.

Tardive Dyskinesia: Biological Mechanisms and Clinical Aspects (#13)
Edited by Marion E. Wolf, M.D., and Aron D. Mosnaim, Ph.D.

Foreword

D r. Carolyn Mazure has edited a most interesting book presenting a fresh look at an old problem, namely—what is the relationship between stress and psychiatric illness? Within this collection of eight chapters, she and the other authors provide a historical context for the study of stress and then present new empirical data on this highly relevant clinical question. The result is an outstanding contribution to clinicians and researchers who want to understand what is known, and what is new, in relation to stress and psychiatric illness.

The diversity of chapters in this book reflects the importance of an interdisciplinary contribution to understanding the relationship between biological and psychosocial dimensions of stress and specific psychiatric illnesses. Even more importantly, the authors of these chapters begin to grapple with the central question of how to integrate multiple variables as well as biological and psychosocial models for understanding the effects of stress. This integrative task is essential in developing a comprehensive explanation for onset or exacerbation of psychiatric illness. Recent work by this author, studying pathways to depression, has suggested biological-genetic models of stress must address at least three separate subtopics: biological clocks or rhythms, the neurobiology of stress, and temperament. It is also clear that concepts of stress physiology and reactivity need to be part of a more extensive examination of stressors associated with the psychosocial-environmental domain.

In this book, we are treated to a variety of conceptual frameworks for studying stressors, ranging from life events models and psychosocial risk factor paradigms to biological challenges for examining stress-related dysregulation of subcortical dopamine activity. We are encouraged to consider initial attempts to bridge the major conceptual gap that currently exists between those investigators who are attempting to examine neurobiological bases of disorders and those investigators who are examining psychosocial theories. This type of hypothesis and strategy development for testing the interrelationships among biological and psychosocial factors uses modern conceptualizations of stressors and is essential to further the field. It is this very interplay among a range of biological and environmental stressors that holds the key to understanding pathways to psychopathology.

The first chapter offers a perceptive historical perspective of the relationship between stress and psychiatric illness and provides a framework for the subsequent chapters. In reviewing the contents of the book, one is immediately struck with the editor's attention to a wide range of psychiatric syndromes in which stress may play a pivotal role, as reflected in well-conceived chapters on schizophrenia, depression, bereavement, posttraumatic stress disorder, and panic disorder. In addition, this book contains an interesting chapter on the relationship of stress to global dysfunctioning, psychopathology, and consequences in the workplace.

Among the major issues identified by each chapter's authors as important to the study of stress is a definitional one: What constitutes stress, and what are the parameters of the definition of a stressor? Interestingly, although investigators are attempting to give full recognition to a range of stressors, it is noteworthy to examine the latest attempt at nosological improvement, that of DSM-IV, in which Axis IV remains an underdeveloped area. The experts who devised DSM-IV accepted that a range of psychosocial or environmental problems may be present that affect the "diagnosis, treatment, and prognosis of mental disorders." They provide a recording form in which relevant types of psychosocial factors can be recorded. Although this may represent a small victory for those interested in stress research, it reflects the secondary role played by stress in our overall understanding of psychiatric disorders. In many ways, as carefully demonstrated in the introductory chapter, the dialogue among the descendants of Kraepelin and Meyer continues. It is our hope that one day there will be a level playing field in terms of operational criteria and expertise that will finally lead to an integrated conceptualization of various types of stressors and their effects. This excellent book is a positive step in the journey toward this goal.

David J. Kupfer, M.D.

Preface

In the clinical setting, it is commonly asked of patients whether there were any events or conditions that preceded the onset of their distress and whether there are continuing or ongoing stressors in their lives. These questions are asked by clinicians based on the belief that events can contribute to the onset of a psychiatric disorder and that stressors can affect the course of disorders. Despite the almost universal acceptance of these notions in clinical care, the systematic study of the relationship of stress to psychiatric illness has been plagued by controversy due to inconsistencies in research results. The aim of this book is to reexamine the purposely provocative question "Does stress cause psychiatric illness?" with new empirical data using contemporary methods and integrative theoretical models. Such data on the role of stressors in psychiatric illness are essential in understanding the etiology of psychopathology and have direct practical applications for treatment and prevention strategies.

In Chapter 1, to provide a context for the seven chapters that follow, Dr. Druss and I render a historical account of when and how stress has been included in theories of mental disorders. We begin with a review of earliest Western writings on mental disorders and trace the evolution of conceptual thinking about psychiatric illness to the present. Theoretical benchmarks that herald major conceptual changes in our understanding of psychiatric illness are noted, and the role of stress in these evolving concepts is provided. The major focus of this chapter, however, is the expansion of knowledge in the twentieth century that fostered the development of psychosocial and biological theories on the relationship of stress and psychiatric illness. We include a review of current nosological, biological, and psychosocial models on the role of stressors in psychiatric illness and discuss some of the major points of contention about the value of each model. We conclude with a call for empirical research and integrative models as a segue to the following chapters.

Four major conceptual approaches to the study of stress and psychiatric illness are reflected in the remaining chapters of this book. First, one can examine the role of stressors in the onset or outcome of a disorder. Based on the idea that stress may play a different role across various disorders, each of four chapters is devoted to the examination of stress in specific psychiatric disorders. The chapters on specific diagnostic categories cover schizophrenia, unipolar and bipolar depression, and panic disorder. Second, one can approach the study of stress and psychiatric illness by examining a disorder in which the experience of stress is central to the diagnosis of the illness. This strategy is exemplified by the chapter on posttraumatic stress disorder. Third, one can examine a condition that is an agreed-on stressor to determine if and when psychiatric illness may result. This is the approach used in the chapter on bereavement and consequent psychiatric illness. Fourth, one can study the effects of stress-reducing interventions on daily functioning and psychiatric disturbance. This is the approach of the final chapter in this book on preventive interventions in the workplace.

Schizophrenia and depression were among the first disorders in which stressors were studied as possible precipitants. The work of Bruce Dohrenwend and colleagues has long been informative in these investigations. In Chapter 2, Dr. Dohrenwend et al. provide an empirical examination of the relationship of stressful life events and other psychosocial risk factors to both schizophrenia and depression. The work presented in this chapter illustrates the importance of considering multiple variables across different domains of psychosocial experience to understand the complex relationship between stressors and illness. Various aspects of recent events, ongoing situations, and personal dispositions are tested in a model designed to identify psychosocial factors that put people at risk for schizophrenia and depression. Results suggest those variables that warrant further investigation in models examining how stress relates to psychiatric illness.

The work of Alan Breier elaborates on the theme set by Dohrenwend et al. by including the examination of biological variables in constructing a stress-diathesis model for schizophrenia. Based on the notion that dysregulation in neurotransmitter systems is more likely to be found under conditions of stress, Dr. Breier presents a creative use of a biological challenge to test a pathophysiologic hypothesis of schizophrenia in Chapter 3. He compares control subjects with patients with schizophrenia to uncover a stress-related deficit in dopamine regulation that appears specific to schizophrenia. Such findings illuminate a biological basis for psychotic illness in the face of stressors.

Although a relationship between depression and antecedent stressors has been consistently found, only a small portion of the variance in depression typically tends to be attributed to stressors. In Chapter 4, to explain more of the variance, Dr. Hammen provides a framework for understanding the complex relationship between stressors and depression and then asks and answers clear and focused questions about specific aspects of this relationship. Methodological refinements illustrated in this chapter include the differentiation of depressed patients into those with bipolar depression and those with unipolar depression, the use of a longitudinal investigation of stressors and depressive onset, and examination of life events in the context of personality variables that may predispose individuals to experience certain types of events as stressors. Most importantly, the data presented in this chapter lend support to the view that there is an interaction between stressors and depression and that stressors occur in stressful contexts that are important targets for clinical intervention.

Historically, the diagnosis of panic disorder requires that at least one panic attack be "spontaneous," that is, not associated with an anxiety-inducing situation. As detailed in Chapter 5 on the relationship of stress to panic, the innovative work of Dr. Falsetti and colleagues suggests a new conceptualization for panic supported by preliminary empirical findings. These authors present the formulation that at least a subset of panic disorder may be precipitated by a traumatic stressor and maintained by subsequent subtle cues that serve as reminders of the stressor, thus generating further attacks. The authors also reconsider the relationship of panic to posttraumatic stress disorder and provide a review of both biological and psychosocial theories that may lend support to their formulation.

As noted earlier, another method for examining the relationship of stress to psychiatric illness is to study a disorder that appears to be caused by a stressor. This is the method used in the work of J. Douglas Bremner and colleagues in their study of posttraumatic stress disorder. Exposure to an experience that would be "markedly distressing to almost anyone" has been central to the diagnosis of posttraumatic stress disorder. However, not everyone exposed to such trauma develops symptoms of this disorder, indicating that exposure to a severe stressor is not the only factor in the etiology of posttraumatic stress disorder. The environmental, neurobiological, and genetic factors that coalesce to precipitate the actual disorder have only begun to be investigated. In Chapter 6, Dr. Bremner et al. outline specific psychosocial and biological prestressor risk factors (e.g., premorbid exposure to other adverse life events, family history of psychiatric illness), peristressor risk factors (e.g., repeated exposure to trauma), and poststressor risk factors (e.g., social support, use of alcohol or drugs) under investigation. They then explain specific hypotheses on the role of these factors in posttraumatic stress disorder. In their empirical work, this research group examines the role of dissociation in the etiology of this disorder and suggests that dissociative responses to trauma are associated with worse outcome, including long-term posttraumatic stress disorder and continued dissociative symptoms. Similar to Dr. Hammen's work on depression, one finding of this group also posits an interactive hypothesis in that posttraumatic stress disorder may set a context for generation of further stress, which contributes to continued psychiatric disturbance.

In Chapter 7, Drs. Kim and Jacobs focus on the experience of loss of a loved one as a universally accepted stressor to examine if and when psychiatric illness may result. In this chapter, normal grief and pathological grief are defined and reviewed, and the process of differentially diagnosing psychiatric disorders during bereavement is explained. With this important and informative groundwork established, the risk factors that contribute to psychiatric disorders with the stress of bereavement can be investigated. These authors then present data that demonstrate bereavement is associated with the onset of psychiatric illness. Specifically, they examine the relationship of pathological grief to major depression, panic, and generalized anxiety disorder and summarize the different risk factors for each of these disorders. Knowledge of such risk factors has clinical implications for understanding complicated bereavement and for guiding interventions. In fact, these authors provide specific information about the use of psychotherapeutic methods and psychotropic drugs in the treatment of complicated bereavement.

In Chapter 8, the final chapter, Drs. Snow and Kline address an essential clinical issue derived from the knowledge that stressors can affect onset of psychiatric illness: whether stress-reducing interventions can affect daily functioning and decrease psychiatric disturbance. The authors review the research literature and assert that work and family stressors are known risk factors for negative physical and mental health outcomes. They present specific models that have been proposed for understanding the effects of stressors and outline the interactional model that best describes the basis for their empirical work. The authors then present longitudinal data from their study on the short- and long-term effects of work-site coping skills interventions on psychological state. Assessment of multiple risk factors as well as of protective factors (such as social support) is emphasized. Results of this work highlight the importance of prevention methodologies that can reduce stressors and the consequent onset of symptomatology.

There is a clear need to supply the clinician and the clinical researcher with information regarding when and how stressors cause or affect the onset and course of psychiatric illness. The authors in this book provide formulations and empirical data that address that need. A variety of disorders are surveyed, and various methods for relating stress to psychiatric illness are provided. The result is a consensus that there is a complex yet increasingly understandable relationship between stress and psychiatric illness.

Carolyn M. Mazure, Ph.D.

Chapter 1

A Historical Perspective on Stress and Psychiatric Illness

Carolyn M. Mazure, Ph.D., and
Benjamin G. Druss, M.D.

Does stress cause psychiatric illness? Throughout Western history, certain traumatic events, such as death of a loved one or the experiences of war, have been recognized as affecting our psychological well-being. However, the relationship between stressful experience and psychiatric illness has only begun to be systematically explicated in the last century.

To trace the role ascribed to stressors in the etiology of mental disorders, we provide a brief historical sketch of how mental illness was understood in Western thinking from Greek times through the nineteenth century. The focus of the chapter, however, is to examine twentieth century notions regarding the relationship between stressful life events and psychiatric illness. As a framework for this examination, we report on how events as stressors have been incorporated into the development of our nosology and into biological and psychosocial explanations of mental illness.

DEFINITION OF TERMS: HISTORICAL ORIGINS OF THE MEANING OF *STRESS*

The word *stress*, of Latin origin, has been a part of the English language since at least the fourteenth century. Its earliest meanings included "hardship, straits, adversity, affliction" as well as the process of using force or pressure on another. The use of the term continued to be broadened to include meanings such as

1

"strain upon endurance" and, even more specifically, "strain upon a bodily organ or a mental power" (Oxford English Dictionary 1989, p. 885). This plurality of definition has continued to date, extends across both common usage and scientific literature, and is highlighted by the observation that the word *stress* has come to be used to describe both a stimulus and a response (Turpin and Lader 1986). We use *stress* as a general term to connote the overall stimulus-response relationship but use *stressor*, the term coined in 1950 by Selye (1956), to mean an outside stimulus acting on an organism. Such stressors can be primarily physical in nature (e.g., pain, infection); however, we concentrate on events as stressors and their relationship to mental disorders.

ROLE OF EVENTS AS STRESSORS IN CONCEPTUALIZATIONS OF MENTAL ILLNESS PRIOR TO THE TWENTIETH CENTURY

Except for certain particular types of traumatic experience, the specific notion that stressful events could affect psychological state was not clearly formulated or well integrated into theories of mental illness until relatively modern times. A multitude of different explanations for illness have acknowledged that environment may have some general effect on mental condition. However, historically, disruption of psychological state was largely attributed to factors ranging from demonic possession to an imbalance in humors, to moral weakness, or to ingestion of toxins. Within this overview, certain individuals are cited as examples of those whose work characterizes an era or are exceptions to it.

Greco-Roman Notions of the Etiology of Illness

The classical Greek view of the cause of illness was based on the humoral theory popularized around 500–400 B.C. by Hippocrates (460–377 B.C.) and other Greek physicians. It suggested that a physical imbalance in one of four bodily humors within the affected individual accounted for physical and mental disease (Ackernecht 1968). The four humors (blood, black bile, yellow bile, and phlegm) were thought to correspond to the elements (air, earth, fire, and water), and it was reasoned by Hippocrates that "if fire should be mastered to a greater extent by the water in the soul, we have then cases of what are called by some 'senseless' people" (Goshen 1967, p. 9). This notion of the mechanism of disease represented a major conceptual advance within Western culture because it replaced prior supernatural traditions with the secular belief that natural phenomena have natural explanations (Alexander and Selesnick 1966).

Direct effects of stressful life events on illness did not clearly play a role in the humoral theory. However, regulation of environmental factors (e.g., air, exercise, food, sleep, and excretions) was acknowledged as having some function in maintaining proper "hygiene" and thus in avoiding disruption of humors (Jackson 1986). Others within the Greco-Roman tradition offered alternative somatic explanations and also acknowledged some general relationship of environmental factors and illness. For example, Soranus of Ephesus, a Roman physician who lived 500 years after Hippocrates (c.A.D. 100), adhered to the naturalistic school of Methodism, which viewed illness as resulting from an abnormal constriction *(status strictus)* or relaxation *(status laxis)* of the solid parts of the body. In terms of mental disorders, Soranus maintained that agitated forms of insanity were caused by excessive constriction, whereas "melancholy" was due to excessive relaxation. He generally allowed that effects of heat, cold, indigestion, drunkenness, insomnia, head trauma, and poisoned food should be incorporated into the larger explanation for illness onset (Goshen 1967). However, despite receiving some acknowledgment, the focus of Greek and Roman physicians was the development of somatically based explanations for illness.

The Middle Ages and the Transition to the Renaissance

The fall of the Roman Empire initiated a return to "supernatural" explanations of psychological disturbance, and the somatic perspective provided by Greco-Roman thought became less prevalent throughout the Middle Ages. During the medieval period, mentally ill persons were often thought to suffer from moral turpitude, believed to be possessed by evil spirits, or thought to be witches or sorcerers who could induce illness in others. Consequently, both somatic contributions and the effects of stressful experience were not included in explanations of mental illness or determination of "treatments," which included exorcism and execution. Introspection, as a method for examining the effects of experience or events on one's psychological life, also was generally unrepresented during the Middle Ages. The writings of St. Augustine (c.a.d. 354–430) provide the classic exception to this general rule. His *Confessions* reflected an attempt to understand experience through self-examination; however, Augustine largely focused on the internal negotiation of inner conflicts rather than on the specific effects of life events on mental disturbance.

Belief in supernatural causation of illness did not come to an abrupt end during the Renaissance. Rather, changes in these notions occurred from the 1300s to 1600s. For instance, Paracelsus (1493–1541), a Swiss-born physician, claimed to reject both the supernatural view held by many clergy and the humoral theory. However, his theories contained elements of each and, in addition, enumerated precipitating factors, including effects of the moon, heredity, poisoned food, and disposition.

> There are four kinds of insane people: Lunatici, Insani, Vesani, and Melancholi. Lunatici are those who get the disease from the moon and react according to it. Insani are those who have been suffering from it since birth and who have brought it from the womb as a family heritage. Vesani are those who have been poisoned and contaminated by food and drink, from which they lose reason and sense. Melancholi are those who by their nature lose their reason and turn insane. (Paracelsus, qtd. in Goshen 1967, p. 51)

The Seventeenth and Eighteenth Centuries

A further reduction in notions of evil spirits and possession as the cause of mental illness occurred during the seventeenth century, despite continued interest in the relationship of the soul to one's general well-being. Most importantly, the "Age of Reason" brought with it a reaffirmation of physiological explanations for illness. Support for the long-held Hippocratic-Galenic humoral theory declined during this era. Instead, body chemical theories, mechanical and hydrodynamic explanations for illness, increased in popularity. A primary role for stressors or life events in the etiology of mental illness was not clearly in evidence within these theories. However, even without benefit of a theory with which to explain the relationship of stressors and illness, there were some who continued to acknowledge the effect of environment on the genesis of illness.

In his well-known work, *The Anatomy of Melancholia*, Robert Burton (1577–1640), an Oxford dean of divinity, noted the role of precipitating factors in the onset of melancholia within his historical account of the description, pathogenesis, and treatment of melancholy. As in Paracelsus' writings, the list of precipitating factors for melancholy included supernatural forces as well as environmental factors such as the heat of the sun, a bad diet, or a blow to the head. Unlike Paracelsus and many earlier theoreticians, Burton also described psychosocial causes for melancholy, including "loss of liberty, servitude, imprisonment, poverty and want, accidents, death of friends" (Burton 1621/1927, p. 110).

The "Enlightenment" that progressed into the eighteenth century was characterized by an emphasis on empirical approaches to the acquisition of knowledge. Advances were being made in various fields of medicine and science using these strategies. Attempts to understand mental disturbance also were being elaborated empirically, and classification systems were becoming more scientifically derived. The work of William Battie (1703–1776), a prominent London physician of the eighteenth century, represents one example of this development. His 1758 book *Treatise on Madness* categorized mental illness into two groups: 1) "original," without organic lesions, and 2) "consequential," following brain disease or injury. Based on his clinical observations, Battie noted that some sources of stress, such as excessive thinking, could bring about an adverse outcome. However, the causes of consequential mental illness were generally limited to somatic factors that included poisons, head trauma, and fevers, and his view took little account of life events or psychosocial factors. As part of this tradition, William Cullen (1712–1790) developed one of the most comprehensive classification systems of this time in which all known diseases were categorized by symptoms, diagnosis, and recommended therapy. Although this work remained focused on physiological cause, Cullen saw the possibility that not all mental illness was decided solely by physiology and introduced the term *neurosis* to mean diseases unaccompanied by fever or localized pathology.

Despite the progress made in furthering a scientific and humane understanding of mental illness, the prevailing view in London during this century was that mental illness was incurable. Battie opposed this position held by John Monro (1715–1791) and others of his family who ran Bethlehem Hospital ("Bedlam") for numerous generations. Monro not only held that "insanity" was incurable, but consequently claimed that there was no point in writing about "madness" or training physicians in the care of the mentally ill. Battie recognized that some patients did recover, and that some improved without treatment or when the contemporary treatment (e.g., bloodletting) was stopped (Hunter and Macalpine 1963).

It was during this period and into the nineteenth century that the initiation of more humane treatment of the mentally ill was rekindled. Asylum inmates began to be differentiated on the basis of whether they were incarcerated for political reasons, for societal crimes, or because they had mental illness. The reform movement of this generation was represented on the European continent and in Great Britain. It also was popularized in the United States by individuals as diverse as Benjamin Rush (1745–1813), who is often spoken of as the father of American psychiatry, and Dorothea Dix (1802–1887), who was the most influential reformer of the nineteenth century and may be considered the mother of humane treatment of the mentally ill in America (Grob 1973).

The Nineteenth Century

A strong descriptive tradition continued, and the development of much of the groundwork for contemporary theories of mental illness occurred during the nineteenth century. Most notably, as notions of etiology were formulated, the relationship between life events as stressors causing or contributing to mental illness increasingly was discussed. One of the most well-known contributors in this regard was Philippe Pinel (1745–1826). It is often cited that Pinel, to ascertain the impact of life events on the onset of mental illness, asked all of his patients whether they had "suffered vexation, grief or reversal of fortune" (qtd. in Rutter 1985, p. 598). In addition to his view that mental illness was the result of heredity and life experiences, Pinel was known for careful observation of symptoms, a belief in the "natural history" of illnesses, and the objective classification of patients. In his work, at Bicêtre (the public hospital for men near Paris) and then at the Salpêtrière (the public hospital for women), he initiated major changes in the treatment of the mentally ill. These changes provided a new perspective on humane treatment and "psychological" treatment of the mentally ill (Weiner 1992).

His student and successor at the Salpétrière, Jean Etienne Esquirol (1772–1840), expanded on Pinel's work in the areas of mental health reform and teaching. He continued the tradition of clinical research and provided information on the epidemiology of patients admitted to the Salpétrière, examining sex, profession, age, prevalence of domestic troubles, "disappointed affection," and physical causes (heredity, head trauma, and intestinal worms). Esquirol also recognized that some phenomena previously thought to be causes of disease, such as use of alcohol, could also be symptoms of an underlying mental illness.

At about the same time, Wilhelm Griesinger (1817–1868), a physician who represented the German emphasis on highly individualized assessment, provided a description of the relationship between stressors and psychiatric illness that is similar to stress-diathesis theories of psychiatric illness found in the latter half of the twentieth century. Griesinger noted that "many individuals live under conditions which are acknowledged to exert a powerful influence on the development of mental diseases, and only a few of them become really insane" (Griesinger 1867/1882, p. 94). He explained this phenomenon in the following manner:

> Commonly the nervous constitution is but a predisposing circumstance, besides which something else is necessary—a real cause,

either a physical disease or a moral influence—in order that the simple disposition may become actual disorder—that the moderate mental aberration may pass into profound insanity, may become an actual cerebral disease. (p. 113)

The influence of societal changes and pressures on the occurrence of mental illness also became a focus of study within the early nineteenth century. This focus resulted in the evolution of social psychiatry (Rosen 1959). This is a discipline that includes in its purview the importance of community experience and events to the psychological state. Amariah Brigham (1798–1849), founder in 1844 of the *American Journal of Insanity*, which was later to become the *American Journal of Psychiatry*, and who was also one of the founders of the American Psychiatric Association, was one of the early proponents of this field of study. One example of some of the early work in this area was Brigham's contention in 1840 in his *Inquiry Concerning the Diseases and Functions of the Brain* that insanity increased due to causes that included the following: "Domestic griefs, Over exertion of mind, Religious anxiety, Political events, Disappointment in love, Disappointed ambition" (qtd. in Hunter and Macalpine 1963, p. 822). This list of experiences provided an indication of the developing emphasis on the relationship of environmental stressors and psychological state.

In these few pages, we have presented a brief overview of the etiology of mental illness, highlighting the role of stressful events in past theories. This outline is in no way meant to be complete, and a thorough review of this history is outside the scope of a single chapter. Nonetheless, as one traces a path of interest in events as stressors leading to illness, it appears that largely up until the nineteenth century, etiological models either did not address the effects of events as stressors affecting the development of mental illness or did so in an indirect, limited, or general way. The twentieth century's explosion of knowledge and theory about psychiatric illness, which resulted in a wider acceptance of the interaction between stressors and psychiatric illness, is now discussed. In a subsequent section of this chapter, we explore how the role of stressors has been incorporated into psychiatric nosology.

PSYCHOSOCIAL STRESSORS AND TWENTIETH–CENTURY NOSOLOGICAL MODELS

This century has seen the continued development of increasingly standardized taxonomies of mental illness. As psychiatric theories have evolved, notions of how to include the influence of psychosocial stressors in these taxonomies have changed along with it.

The contemporary classifications of mental illness that best illustrate this issue are characterized by three approaches. The first of these approaches is exemplified by the work of Emil Kraepelin, who acknowledged but deemphasized stressors. He favored a descriptive approach to psychiatric disorders and believed them to be organic in etiology. The second approach is characterized by the perspective of Adolf Meyer, who asserted that the description of a disease entity was incomplete without an understanding of the psychosocial context. The third approach is that seen in the multiaxial system of the *Diagnostic and Statistical Manual of Mental Disorders* (DSM), which largely continues in the Kraepelinian tradition but also attempts to identify psychosocial stressors. In the following sections, we explore the treatment of psychosocial stressors in twentieth-century psychiatric taxonomy by noting the contributions of Kraepelin and Meyer, and then focus on the evolution of the DSM in the United States.

Emil Kraepelin

Emil Kraepelin (1856–1926) created a classification of illness that has provided the basis for most twentieth-century taxonomic models (Blashfield 1984). He was strongly influenced by teachers such as Wilhelm Wundt, one of the first experimental psychologists who emphasized empiricism and observation. Kraepelin maintained that view when he moved from the psychology laboratory to the German asylums and when he began to assemble his *Compendium of Psychiatry* in 1883, with further editions published under the title *A Short Textbook of Psychiatry*, and finally *A Textbook of Psychiatry*. Kraepelin's textbook, from its first edition in 1883 until the 9th edition published posthumously in 1927, reflected his conceptualization of mental illnesses as organic disease entities (Menninger 1963). He is best known for his contributions in the 5th and 6th editions, which provided a delineation of two major categories of psychiatric illness: manic-depressive psychosis and dementia praecox. He emphasized the role of illness course in distinguishing between these two entities because "very similar symptoms can at first glance, be apparent in the course of very different diseases" (Kraepelin 1904, qtd. in Blashfield 1984, p. 14).

Although he described the role of heredity, fevers, and childbearing as, at times, preceding these illnesses, he deemphasized the role of life events in influencing the course of these illnesses. "We must regard all alleged injuries as possibly sparks for the discharge of individual attacks, but . . . the real cause of the malady must be sought in permanent internal changes . . . which are innate" (Kraepelin 1921, qtd. in Post 1992, p. 999). Kraepelin further described illness as progressing according to the underlying biology of the disease, and he focused on whether the disease had a deteriorating course ("dementia praecox") or not ("manic-depressive psychosis").

Adolf Meyer

Adolf Meyer (1866–1950), European born and trained, was originally attracted to Kraepelin's work and played an important role in bringing that work to the United States. However, he gradually became disenchanted with the utility of classification systems, asserting that such systems were, by necessity, overly reductionistic. He also rejected the notion that an underlying biological etiology was the sole, or even essential, precipitant to psychiatric illness. Instead, he emphasized the overriding importance of psychosocial stressors in determining the genesis and course of psychiatric disorders and maintained that stressors were inextricably linked to any underlying biological disease entity. In describing a case of depression, he noted that

the aetiology thus involves: (1) constitutional make-up and (2) a precipitating factor. . . . It is my contention that we must use both facts and that, of the two, . . . the precipitating factor is of the

greater importance because it alone gives us an idea of the actual
defect and a suggestion as to how to strengthen the person so that
he may become resistive. (Meyer 1908, qtd. in Cooper 1986, p. 19)

Adolf Meyer developed a theory of "psychobiology," which
emphasized the interdependence of biology, psychology, events,
and social environment in shaping mental illness. He characterized psychiatric disorders as "reaction sets," clusters of signs and
symptoms arising in the context of life stressors. He saw such
illnesses as failures to adapt to stressors (Blashfield 1984). His
psychobiology replaced the Kraepelinian focus on classification
and emphasized context as well as treatment and prevention of
psychiatric illness.

Evolution of the *Diagnostic and Statistical Manual of Mental Disorders*

The development of the *Diagnostic and Statistical Manual of Mental
Disorders* was in response to the need for a uniform nomenclature
that would also address some of the problems of the existing
taxonomies. A review of the development of DSM also highlights
how contemporary American psychiatry has regarded the possible contribution of psychosocial stressors to the onset and exacerbation of mental illness.

There have been five DSM editions published by the American
Psychiatric Association: DSM-I (1952), DSM-II (1968), DSM-III
(1980), DSM-III-R (1987), and DSM-IV (1994). DSM-I was influenced by the theoretical perspective of Adolf Meyer in that the
term *reaction* was used throughout the DSM-I classification, reflecting Meyer's view that "mental disorders represented reactions of the personality to psychological, social, and biological
factors" (American Psychiatric Association 1987, p. xviii).

In contrast, DSM-II used diagnostic terms that generally did
not imply a particular theoretical framework. This edition was
based on and was an attempt to be compatible with the mental
disorders section of the 8th edition of the *International Classification of Diseases* (ICD-8; World Health Organization 1968). This
move represented a shift from a Meyerian perspective to a more
Kraepelinian one, an attempt to categorize mental illnesses as

discrete entities independent of their psychosocial contexts (Millon 1986).

DSM-III maintained the generally atheoretical approach of DSM-II but was a major revision in that it represented a reaffirmation of the descriptive tradition, expanding descriptions considerably and adding diagnostic criteria. Among the other major changes was the inclusion of a multiaxial system of classification. There had been interest in multidimensional evaluation for a long time within psychiatry (Williams 1985). By the mid-1970s, as drafts of DSM-III were being organized by the American Psychiatric Association DSM-III Task Force on Nomenclature and Statistics, interest began to take form with specific proposals for possible multiaxial systems. As a result of the considerable support for such a system expressed during this time, and, in particular, at a 1976 conference to examine the progress of DSM-III's formulation, the task force and its consultants incorporated the current multiaxial approach to diagnosis. This was done to provide a better representation of the relationship among biological, psychological, and social aspects of mental disorders. Of additional note is the fact that this edition was not based on the 9th revision of the *International Classification of Diseases* (ICD-9; World Health Organization 1979), which was also being prepared at that same time, because ICD-9 was not judged to be sufficiently detailed for clinical and research use in the United States.

Most authors concur that the addition of Axis IV (severity of psychosocial stressors) represented a significant, if imperfect, improvement in accounting for the impact of psychosocial forces on mental illness. Millon (1986), one of the members of the DSM-III task force, noted that

> the official recognition that psychosocial environments play a role in the development and exacerbation of mental disorders, though patently obvious, is nevertheless an achievement of great import. Not only does it acknowledge the empirical fact that disturbances that arise in response to stressors have better prognoses than those that do not, but, more impressively, it signifies in an officially recorded fashion the realization that psychosocial factors establish a context within which disorders not only unfold, but are sustained and exacerbated. (p. 56)

There was considerable debate during the formulation of DSM-III about the most useful way to organize the assessment of psychosocial stressors. This debate resulted in the conclusions that 1) there was insufficient information available to construct a rating system that assessed all aspects of the stress process, 2) a complex system of rating life events was not practical because users were already overburdened with learning the complexities of DSM-III, and 3) an objective characterization of stressor severity should be used (Williams 1985). Consequently, a global rating of etiologically significant stressors was adopted with examples of how to rate stressor severity based on the reaction of an "average person."

One of the first major issues that subsequently arose was whether this axis would be used consistently by different raters. In reviewing the interrater reliability studies on DSM-III Axis IV, Skodol and Shrout (1989) concluded that Axis IV ratings were shown to have at least "limited reliability," but the number of available studies was small.

A second major issue was whether DSM-III Axis IV was a valid measure of stressor severity. Five of the six studies that addressed this concern compared the relationship of Axis IV ratings either with patient variables or with outcome variables that were thought to be associated with high versus low stress.

Zimmerman et al. (1985) predicted that high Axis IV ratings would be correlated with nonendogenous depression and low Axis IV ratings with endogenous depression. They found that high ratings correlated with increased familial rates of alcoholism, increased rates of personality disorder, increased suicide attempts, and increased morbid risk of depression, whereas low ratings correlated with dexamethasone suppression test nonsuppression and increased age. The authors concluded that these findings generally supported the validity of Axis IV. Similarly, Schrader et al. (1986) found lower Axis IV ratings in patients with endogenous depression than in patients with reactive depression. Patients with organic psychiatric disorders also tended to have lower ratings than psychotic or nonpsychotic patients; patients with nonaffective psychoses were judged as having lower Axis IV ratings than those patients with affective psychoses.

Mezzich et al. (1984) found a low yet significant positive correlation between Axis IV ratings and the decision to hospitalize a patient. However, these authors indicated that Axis IV added little to the prediction of whether the outcome was hospitalization when considered in conjunction with Axis V (global assessment of functioning) ratings. Gordon et al. (1985) hypothesized that hospital length of stay is increased by level of stressors but decreased by higher levels of functioning. They reported a significant relationship between a "strain ratio" (Axis IV score/rescaled Axis V score) and inpatient length of stay.

Zimmerman et al. (1987) examined whether DSM-III Axis IV ratings predicted outcome in depressed inpatients. The authors found that higher Axis IV ratings were associated with increased depressive symptoms at discharge but that current ratings did not predict outcome at 6 months.

In a more traditional approach to determining construct validity, Skodol and Shrout (1989) compared DSM-III Axis IV ratings with severity of psychosocial stressors, as measured using the Psychiatric Epidemiology Research Interview. DSM-III Axis IV ratings correlated significantly with the interview ratings that assessed event-related change and disruption. However, these authors found that DSM-III's requirement that an event have etiological significance in the initiation or worsening of a disorder for it to be judged a stressor led to discrepancies in the assessment of Axis IV.

With the publication of DSM-III-R, this requirement of etiological significance was broadened to include those events that may have contributed to illness onset or exacerbation. It has yet to be tested whether this change would have affected interrater agreement or measures of validity.

Although some of the problems inherent in the quantification of psychosocial stressors have been outlined in criticisms of DSM-III-R Axis IV, there is no ideal methodology for measuring stressors, particularly in a cross-sectional or retrospective evaluation. DSM-IV, published in 1994, retains the Axis IV recording of "problems" or stressors. However, there are a number of changes in how these are coded. First, rating of severity of stressors has been eliminated. The sample Multiaxial Evaluation Form (American Psychiatric Association 1994, p. 34) contains a checklist for specifying problems across nine possible categories of life experience without any ranking of magnitude. Second, there is no distinction made between acute and chronic problems or stressors. Third, problems can be listed that may have contributed to the initiation or exacerbation of a disorder as well as problems that are a consequence of an individual's psychopathology. This represents a continued shift away from attempts to identify etiologically significant stressors.

Other Classification Methods

Other classification methods, such as quantitative approaches, have also enjoyed popularity and contributed to the organization of psychiatric phenomenology and nosology (Blashfield 1984; Grove and Andreasen 1986). These statistical techniques have largely focused on the aggregation of symptoms to formulate diagnoses but do not theoretically preclude use of other types of data, such as presence of stressful events, in segregating groups of patients. Consequently, these methods may hold increased promise for future taxonomies because they need not be bound to a single model of mental illness.

ROLE OF STRESSORS IN CONTEMPORARY BIOLOGICAL MODELS OF PSYCHIATRIC ILLNESS

Biologically oriented psychiatry has sought to understand the pathophysiological mechanisms underlying mental illness and to identify the variables that may initiate the biological events associated with illness onset. The last 20 years, in particular, have seen the development of theoretical model-building and empirical studies in this area. This work has included an exploration of the physiology of the stress response and its relationship to psychiatric illness.

Stress-Diathesis Models of Mental Illness

Stress-diathesis models of psychiatric illness propose a preexisting, often inherited, disposition or "vulnerability" for an illness.

These models hypothesize that the illness becomes manifest when a vulnerable individual is exposed to a particular type of "triggering" event or stressor. Although the idea of a stress-vulnerability model is not exclusive to the twentieth century (e.g., Griesinger 1867/1882), contemporary models have become more sophisticated and have focused on specific illnesses—particularly schizophrenia (Meehl 1962; Spring and Coons 1982; Zubin and Spring 1977) and depression (Monroe and Simons 1991). In the following segments of this section, we address the evolving biological conceptualizations of the interaction of vulnerability, stressors, and psychiatric illness.

Vulnerability

An individual's vulnerability to develop a psychiatric illness is likely to be a function of a variety of factors. Genetics almost certainly plays an important role in determining vulnerability to most major psychiatric disorders. Family studies, twin studies, adoption studies, and, more recently, molecular genetic mapping techniques have indicated that genetic loading is likely a risk factor for schizophrenia (e.g., Guze et al. 1983; Kendler et al. 1985; Kety 1983; McGue et al. 1983; Tsuang et al. 1980), affective disorders (e.g., Egeland et al. 1987; Mendlewicz and Rainer 1977; Wender et al. 1986), and anxiety disorders (e.g., Torgersen 1983). However, as Egeland et al. (1987) point out, "Not all who inherit the gene will manifest the illness" (p. 328).

Other nongenetic factors operating via physiological mechanisms, such as in utero injury, viral infection, diet (Wender et al. 1986), or drug use (Bowers et al. 1990), may also create vulnerability to illness later in life. Evidence of such nongenetic factors may include radionucleotide studies of cerebral blood flow in monozygotic twins discordant for schizophrenia, which have found relative hypofrontality in affected twins (Berman et al. 1992; Weinberger et al. 1992).

It has been hypothesized that early psychological trauma may affect physiology and induce chronic biological vulnerability to certain psychiatric illnesses. For instance, Breier et al. (1988) pointed out that early loss has been associated with enduring neurobiological alterations in nonhuman animal studies. Their findings in humans indicate that neuroendocrine alterations in the hypothalamic-pituitary-adrenal axis were associated with poorer quality of childhood home life and adaptation after parental loss in those adults with psychopathology compared with those without psychiatric illness who also experienced early loss. Occurrence of illness also may make an individual more susceptible to recurrences of illness. Post (1992) suggested that sensitization to psychosocial stressors and to episode occurrence affects physiology at the level of gene expression, making individuals more vulnerable to subsequent stressors and episodes of illness. Finally, vulnerability has also been hypothesized to be a function of the absence of protective psychosocial buffers, such as a social support network (Rutter 1985) or cognitive strategies for coping (Monroe and Simons 1991).

Hans Selye and the Development of Biological Models of Stress Research

In the early part of the century, physiological psychologists who were developing theories of emotion were studying the effects of both physical and psychological stressors on laboratory animals. For example, in 1911, Walter Cannon performed experiments exposing cats to barking dogs and showed that nonphysical stressors could be potent stimuli for evoking physiological reactions, "in particular the release of what later appeared to be catecholamines by the adrenal medulla" (Vingerhoets 1985, p. 2). Cannon described such stressors as disruptions to an organism's "homeostasis" (a term coined by him) and described the "fight or flight" stress response as an organism's attempt to regain equilibrium. As Mason (1975a) pointed out, Cannon even proposed the concept of "critical stress levels," that is, "those capable of inducing a breaking strain in the homeostatic mechanisms" (p. 7).

On the heels of this seminal work, Hans Selye's research provided what one author has called the foundation on which modern biological stress research has been built (Vingerhoets 1985). In a brief article in *Nature* published in 1936, Selye first described the "general adaptation syndrome." This phenomenon, which he had observed in animal studies, appeared to represent a nonspecific response of the body to a variety of noxious agents. He delineated three phases of the stress response: 1) the "alarm reaction," the organism's initial biological mobilization in response to a stressor; 2) the stage of resistance during which the organism must adapt and restore depleted reserves; and 3) the stage of exhaustion after prolonged exposure to a noxious stimulus when the organism can no longer successfully adapt to the stressor (Selye 1956). Throughout his later work, Selye emphasized the notion that this stress response was a uniform, nonspecific response to a wide variety of different stressors (Mason 1975a). He also later made clear that

> not all states of stress, or threatened homeostasis, were noxious. . . . Hence, he believed that mild, brief, and controllable states of challenged homeostasis could actually be perceived as pleasant or exciting and could be positive stimuli to emotional and intellectual growth and development. (qtd. in Chrousos and Gold 1992, p. 1245)

The area of stress physiology was dominated by the creative concepts of Hans Selye for several decades, but his work was not without its critics. For example, John Mason, a stress physiologist, performed empirical studies that called into question two notions central to Selye's theory (Mason 1971, 1975b). First, he showed that emotional arousal provided the crucial immediate step linking stressors and the stress response and that such responses were likely organized at a higher, "psychological" level of organization than Selye had described. Second, he questioned the notion of nonspecificity of the general adaptation syndrome, postulating that organisms respond to different stressors with different neuroendocrine responses. In support of this second hypothesis, he found characteristic patterns of hormonal response to specific stressors when he examined multihormonal profiles (Mason 1975b).

Both Selye's and Mason's work emphasized the connection between stressors and an organism's neurohormonal state. Other investigators following in this tradition have provided research that supports the fundamental notion that psychological as well as physical stressors can differentially affect a variety of hormones of the neuroendocrine system (Vingerhoets 1985).

Advances in the psychoneuroendocrinology of stress were limited by technical difficulties in identifying, isolating, and localizing hormones. As Mason (1971) pointed out, "Prior to 1950, the study of endocrine regulation was based largely on relatively indirect and nonspecific methods, such as glandular weight, glandular histology, bioassays, or the metabolic effects of hormones" (p. 323). After 1950, new analytic techniques for biochemical measurement, such as chromatography, immunoassay, and microspectrophotometry, greatly advanced biological stress research. Rapid advances in this area of neurohormonal measurement techniques were generally seen again in the 1970s. For example, radioimmunoassays sensitive enough to measure prolactin reliably in human plasma were developed. Also, by the 1970s, psychobiological models were becoming increasingly multifactorial with increased interest in catecholamines and disrupted behavior. The work of Akiskal and McKinney (1973), for example, proposed the integration of findings from genetic research, animal studies on early loss, data on "learned helplessness" induced by uncontrollable stress, and the effects of biogenic amines on behavior in formulating a biologically based stress-diathesis model for depression. These authors then presented a model suggesting the importance of chemical, experiential, and behavioral variables in understanding depression (Akiskal and McKinney 1975). Rather than exclusively examining life events as direct precipitants to illness, Akiskal (1982) also focused on the possible causal effects of life events on vulnerability.

Current Neurobiological Models: Stressors, Stress Response, and Psychiatric Illness

Current research supports Selye's basic notion of a generalized stress response in that "both physical and emotional stressors set into motion central and peripheral responses to preserve homeostasis" (Chrousos and Gold 1992, p. 1245). Such a response is accompanied by elevated heart rate, blood pressure, and respiratory rate and generates increased alertness and vigilance. There is a concurrent decrease in feeding, reproduction, and immune response. In answer to an appropriate threat, and as a time-limited reaction, this stress response is adaptive and self-preservative. However, animal studies have found that inescapable stress adversely alters brain norepinephrine and serotonin levels (Glavin 1985; Weiss et al. 1970) and α_2-receptor regulation (Birch et al. 1986). Packan and Sapolsky (1990) described the potential for glucocorticoids secreted under excessive or prolonged stress to potentiate destruction of hippocampal neurons.

The two primary components central to the stress response appear to be neurons that produce and release corticotropin-releasing hormone (CRH) and the locus coeruleus–norepinephrine system (Chrousos and Gold 1992; Gold et al. 1988). The former system, with neuronal cell bodies primarily localized in the paraventricular nucleus of the hypothalamus, and the latter, located in the brain stem, can both enhance arousal and increase anxiety. The two systems also stimulate each other in a positive feedback loop. They are thought to activate regions of the brain involved with cognition (prefrontal cortex), motivation and reinforcement (nucleus accumbens), and emotional modulation (amygdala). At the same time, they inhibit the reproductive axis, the growth axis, and the inflammatory immune response.

Chrousos and Gold (1992) postulated that although activation of the CRH/locus coeruleus–norepinephrine systems may be adaptive on an acute basis, chronic activation of these systems may result in pathophysiology that induces the symptoms seen in psychiatric illness. They hypothesized that illnesses induced in this fashion can be divided into two categories. The first category includes those illnesses associated with increased CRH secretion and consequent chronic overactivation of the "stress system" (e.g., melancholic depression, panic disorder, and obsessive-compulsive disorder). The second category includes illnesses associated with decreased CRH secretion (e.g., atypical depression, chronic fatigue syndrome) and other disorders characterized by pathologic hypoarousal. These authors also postulated that an individual's inherent sensitivity to stressors may represent a vulnerability that results in a predisposition to a pathologically hyperactive or hypoactive state. This biological "sensitivity" could result from a "genetic defect in metabolism" or may be acquired as a result of a critical event such as early loss or separation. Ultimately, this model, as well as other biological stress-diathesis models, requires a vulnerability in combination with a stressor of appropriate type, duration, and magnitude.

Other work has also linked stress-related dysregulation of specific neurochemical axes with particular psychiatric illnesses. For example, Deutch et al. (1990) used an animal model to investigate possible stress-induced dopamine changes in animals with prefrontal lesions. They reasoned that the prefrontal cortical dysfunction found in schizophrenia may be represented by prefrontal lesions in rats. Their work has shown that mild stress increased mesolimbic dopamine in rats with lesioned prefrontal neurons but not in rats without such lesions. This type of finding may provide a partial explanation as to why stressors can cause an exacerbation of psychotic symptoms in those patients with schizophrenia who have prefrontal cortical dysfunction.

Others have begun to generate models for understanding biochemical changes during depression by linking observed neurobiological changes during stress to the known action of antidepressants. Hyman and Nestler (1993) noted the centrality of the hypothalamic-pituitary axis, as well as the serotonergic and noradrenergic neuronal systems, in the stress response. They pointed out that these same systems are primary targets of antidepressants. For instance, they indicated that stress can produce sustained increases in locus coeruleus (noradrenergic) firing and tyrosine hydroxylase expression, effects that are reversed by chronic antidepressant administration.

As previously noted, Post (1992) proposed a detailed biogenetic hypothesis in which psychosocial stressors might lead to depression. He suggested that stressors result in the induction of the proto-oncogene *c-fos,* which activates a cascade of neurobiological events. Some of these effects may be lasting. Such long-term effects may produce "kindling" in which each recurrent bout of depression requires a less significant stressor, and ultimately such episodes occur autonomously.

Given the relatively limited knowledge about the neurobiology of mental illness, as well as about the precise nature of the physiological underpinnings of the stress response, attempts to link the two are still incomplete. Nonetheless, hypothesized links provide an interesting glimpse into a future where greater knowledge of the interaction of neurobiology with environment may provide us with a better understanding of how to treat and, possibly, to prevent mental illness.

ROLE OF STRESSORS IN PSYCHOLOGICAL AND PSYCHOSOCIAL MODELS OF MENTAL DISORDERS

Traumatic or stressful events have played a significant role in most psychological theories on the evolution of disturbed mood, cognition, or behavior. Perhaps the best example of a psychological theory that incorporates reaction to traumatic events as fundamental to explanations of psychological disturbance is psychoanalytic theory. The work of Sigmund Freud (1856–1939) profoundly influenced the way that modern psychiatry and psychology viewed the effects of stressful events on an individual. For instance, in "Mourning and Melancholia," Freud contrasted the process of mourning, an individual's response to the death of a loved one, to melancholia that "is in some way related to an object-loss which is withdrawn from consciousness, in contradistinction to mourning, in which there is nothing about the loss that is unconscious" (Freud 1917/1957). In "Anxiety and Instinctual Life," Freud explicated the role of early "traumatic moments" in producing anxiety in later life:

> The object of the anxiety, is invariably the emergence of a traumatic moment, which cannot be dealt with by the rules of the pleasure principle. . . . [there is] a twofold origin of anxiety—one as a direct consequence of the traumatic moment and the other as a signal threatening repetition of such a moment. (Freud 1933/1965, p. 95)

Subsequent psychological models have differed from psychoanalytic theory in the explanation of psychological disturbance. However, stressful events continue to play a pivotal role in many contemporary models. For instance, cognitive therapy emphasizes the importance of presently held cognitive patterns through which an individual interprets life events, and maintains that analysis of events and experiences is central to the therapy (Haaga et al. 1991).

Inherent in the evolution of most psychological treatment models is the notion that it is more important to understand the perceived meaning of an event than to determine the exact nature of an occurrence. Within that tradition, Lazarus proposed a "transactional" model of life events and psychological disturbance that involves a complex reciprocal relationship between events and a variety of processes particular to an individual:

> Our theory holds that psychological stress is determined by the person's appraisal of a specific encounter with the environment; this appraisal is shaped by person factors including commitments, vulnerabilities, beliefs, and resources and by situation factors including the nature of the threat, its imminence, and so on. (Lazarus and Folkman 1984, p. 289)

From this list of potential factors that may influence the impact of stressors, a number of investigators postulated that in terms of psychosocial variables, an individual's coping skills and social support recruitment, in particular, can either accentuate or diminish the effect of life events. Coping has been defined as a mechanism "that protects people from being psychologically harmed by problematic social experience" (Pearlin and Schooler 1978, p. 2). Types of coping include cognitive and behavioral strategies for reducing the impact of stressors. Examination of coping styles in those persons with schizophrenia or with depression suggests that coping is at least different from that in control subjects and probably less effective (Barnett and Gotlib 1988; Lukoff et al. 1984). It is unknown if such coping styles precede the onset of illness or result from the disorder. Assessment of coping in long-term follow-up of unipolar depressive patients has shown a positive effect of problem-solving and affective-regulation forms of coping on both role functioning and symptom expression (Swindle et al. 1989), particularly in times of high stress (Holahan and Moos 1991).

The term *social network* is usually used to refer to an individual's connections with family, friends, coworkers, and neighbors (Flaherty et al. 1983). Some research has suggested that patients with effective social support systems have decreased rates and severity of psychiatric illness in the face of stressors (e.g., Brown and Harris 1978; Flaherty et al. 1983). Aneshensel and Stone (1982) and Cohen and Wills (1985) indicated that in addition to buffering the effects of stressful events, social networks also may directly ameliorate depressive symptomatology. However, the mechanisms through which social networks either buffer the onset or diminish the severity of psychiatric illness remain unclear.

In reference to the relationship of life events and psychiatric illness, contemporary psychosocial research largely has focused on determining the unique contribution of recent independent life events to illness onset or exacerbation. In this portion of the chapter, we focus on the empirical studies designed to examine this issue. We provide a brief summary of the literature on schizophrenia and depression because these two syndromes have been the most commonly investigated. Finally, we discuss the development of instruments for assessing stressors and present some of the major methodological issues in assessment of life events.

Relationship of Life Events to Onset of Illness in Schizophrenia

Brown and Birley (1968) provided one of the earliest, and now most frequently cited, studies indicating a positive relationship between life events and episode onset in schizophrenia. In a sample of 50 patients hospitalized for a first episode or recurrence of schizophrenia, the authors found that 46% had experienced at least one "independent" major life event in the 3 weeks prior to onset, whereas only 14% of control subjects had experienced such an event 3 weeks prior to interview. The rate of independent life events did not differ between patients and control subjects in the previous 13 weeks. Independent events were those "imposed on the patient . . . [and that were] outside" the patient's control and not brought on by the patient's "unusual" behavior (p. 205). According to the authors, these findings provided initial support for the notion that recent events could precipitate an episode of illness, although they maintained that events were not a sufficient cause for onset. Later, Brown considered that a better representation of the effect of life events was one in which events were simply facilitating a process already underway (Brown and Harris 1978).

A limited number of subsequent retrospective case-control studies and prospective studies have continued to explore this relationship. Review of this literature has led some authors to conclude that there is some association of life events to onset or relapse in schizophrenic illness (e.g., Day et al. 1987; Lukoff et al. 1984). Others (e.g., Dohrenwend et al. 1992) noted inconsistencies between studies and methodological flaws within studies that continue to make it difficult to draw definitive conclusions as to the strength of such a relationship.

There are a number of factors that make the study of recent life events in schizophrenia particularly challenging. First, it can be difficult even to determine the occurrence of recent independent events. Both initial episodes and relapses of schizophrenia can have an insidious onset in which less obvious psychotic symptoms precede the onset of overt psychosis. Thus, it is not always easy to determine whether occurrence of stressors is in fact "independent" or a function of the patient's incipient illness. Retrospective reports of events can also be affected by current state or recall. This issue has led researchers to suggest the value of considering prospective designs in studying life events. It has also been suggested that individuals with the disorder may have other attributes that put them at higher risk for relapse. For example, patients with schizophrenia who have families with high levels of expressed emotion may have sufficient chronic stress to elicit exacerbations without acute stressors (Leff and Vaughn 1980).

It has also been suggested that the methodology for these studies must continue to be refined in terms of ascertaining other possible risk factors such as family history of disorder, as well as distinguishing between first-episode index cases and recurrent ones, assessing severity of symptoms (particularly mood) at time of interview, and clarifying further an objective scale for rating severity of events (Dohrenwend et al. 1992).

Determination of whether patients are stabilized on neuroleptic medication may also influence the impact of psychosocial stressors. In a well-designed prospective study, Ventura et al. (1992) showed that patients with schizophrenia who were medicated had a greater incidence of independent life events preceding exacerbations than did those patients not receiving medication. This finding is consistent with earlier observations (Birley and Brown 1970; Leff et al. 1973) and the hypothesis (Leff 1987) that maintenance medication raises a patient's threshold to relapse, thus decreasing the probability of an episode of illness unless one is exposed to significant stressors. Conversely, unmedicated patients may be so vulnerable to illness that an acute life event is not necessary to trigger an exacerbation of their illness.

Relationship of Life Events to Onset of Illness in Depression

A number of studies, both retrospective (Paykel 1979) and prospective (Brown et al. 1987; Lewinsohn et al. 1988), have found a relationship between stressful life events and the onset of depression (for an extensive review, see Monroe and Depue 1991). In comparing the incidence of independent life events prior to depression with control subjects during a comparable period, Brown and Harris (1978) demonstrated higher rates of severely stressful events in depressed patients prior to onset compared with control subjects. In investigating the same issue, Shrout et al. (1989) identified 12 events that appeared independent of a respondent's psychiatric status, such as "being laid off because of a workforce reduction." These events were considered independent or "fateful" (i.e., ones in which the individual did not participate), whereas "being fired" would be nonfateful (i.e., a consequence of a person's actions). Their findings suggested that fateful events were 2.5 times more frequent in those who had depressive illness than in community control subjects.

Although a general consensus exists that stressors play a role in the development of depressive disorder, questions remain about the magnitude of that effect and the universality of stressors as a causal agent. Not all depressions are preceded by detectable stressors, and certainly major life events frequently occur without subsequent depressions. Consequently, a number of models, including stress-diathesis theories, have been proposed to explain the relationship between stressors and depression. These theories acknowledge the importance of other variables, both psychosocial and biological, in predicting illness onset or exacerbation. This acknowledgment has also led to refinement in the way in which this issue has been investigated.

For example, it has been hypothesized that in any one patient the relationship of life events to depression may differ from first depressive episode to later episodes. In reviewing this literature, Post (1992) proposed that life events are less influential in subsequent episodes of depression because initial depressive episodes make individuals more sensitive to recurrent depressions. This kindling model predicts that although first episodes would tend to be associated with life events, later depressions will be more autonomous and hence unrelated to external stressors. In support of this hypothesis, Post cited a number of studies such as that by Ezquiaga et al. (1987), who found that life events were significantly more likely to occur in patients with first- or second-episode unipolar depressions than in those with recurrent unipolar depression. These investigators also found that patients experiencing recurrent depressions were no more likely to have experienced life events than were control patients from a surgical trauma service. These results have been supported by findings from other studies of unipolar depression (Cassano et al. 1989; Dolan et al. 1985; Ghaziuddin et al. 1990), although these studies did not include a comparison control group.

In contrast, some research has found little (Perris 1984) or no (Bidzinska 1984) difference between the impact of life events on first-episode and recurrent unipolar depressions. Other investigators found an inverse relationship between episode number and life events for manic episodes (Ambelas 1979, 1987) and for bipolar depressions (Bidzinska 1984; Cassano et al. 1989).

Other work examined whether depression can be divided into subtypes based on the occurrence of life events prior to onset of illness. Bebbington et al. (1988) and Katschnig et al. (1986) called the prototypical endogenous/exogenous distinction into question, noting that in patients with severe depression, the incidence of preceding life events was equal to that in patients with milder "neurotic" depressions.

Life events preceding, during, or after an acute episode may also have an impact on the course of depression. Findings from

Miller et al. (1987) suggest that stressors of "uncertain outcome" may predict depressive episodes of longer duration. Stressors that occur during a depression have been found to be associated with exacerbations of symptoms (Brown and Harris 1978) and with decreased tricyclic antidepressant response (Lloyd et al. 1981). Monroe et al. (1983) found that a greater number of life events preceding a depression predicted greater likelihood of enhanced recovery for a sample of unipolar depressed female outpatients. Stressful life events occurring after resolution of an episode of major depression also have been shown to predict relapse (Paykel and Tanner 1976). It also has been hypothesized that for an event to affect an individual adversely, its characteristics may have to correspond to particular vulnerabilities in that person (Hammen et al. 1989; Segal et al. 1992). Finally, the occurrence of depression may create interpersonal conditions that generate more stressors. Hammen (1991) reported that in a 1-year longitudinal study of women with unipolar depression compared with control subjects, those with recurrent depression had higher rates of dependent or nonfateful life events that in turn might induce further depressive symptomatology.

Measurement of Recent Life Events

Among the reasons why it has been difficult to incorporate the effect of stressful life events into a model explaining the onset or exacerbation of psychiatric disorders is the problem of establishing an assessment method. To illustrate this point, we discuss three of the major methodological issues in stress assessment.

One of the first issues to arise in life event measurement has been whether to devise an objective scale for rating stressor severity or to use subjective reports of event magnitude. As Lazarus and Folkman (1984) argued, effects of an event depend on how an individual appraises the significance of the event (i.e., what the outcome of the event will mean). It has been reasoned that an individual's perception is more clinically useful than an objective assessment because subjective reports reflect the patient's vulnerability and, thus, are more closely tied to individual outcome. In fact, this may be accurate on an individual basis (Dohrenwend et al. 1978). However, it has been argued that such a measure, due to its dependence on the personality and behavior of the individual, confounds the independent assessment of stressor severity with the outcome. This issue became a salient one in the formulation of the DSM-III Axis IV. The American Psychiatric Association Task Force on Nomenclature and Statistics concluded that an objective characterization of stressors was necessary, or Axis IV might become a reflection of individual psychopathology rather than of psychosocial stressors. At this juncture, there appears to be general agreement that objective ratings are necessary in studying the independent contribution of life events; however, some investigators still maintain that perceived stress is important in predicting outcome (Cohen and Wills 1985).

A second major assessment debate has centered on the value of life event checklists designed to rate the presence or absence of a finite number of events versus a semistructured interview that allows for a more broad and detailed report of events. The checklist method is often characterized by the work of Holmes and Rahe (1967) in the form of the Schedule of Recent Events, later revised to be the Social Readjustment Rating Scale. This work played a formative role in the development of life event scales by objectifying the amount of social readjustment associated with prototypically stressful events. It set down an empirically derived list of potentially stressful events, with consensually derived, a priori agreement about the magnitude of social change associated with a given event.

However, this technique was not without drawbacks. Checklist items (e.g., change in financial state, minor violations in the law, change in the health of a family member) were not considered precise descriptions of events. As Paykel (1983) pointed out, although the checklist technique could be used without rater bias and without the confound of a subjective report, it was "a blunt tool" in that it could overlook the particular circumstances of individual event occurrences.

As other checklists measuring change or distress associated with events appeared, other investigators developed semi-structured interviews that included probe questions permitting additional detail for rating events. Representative work includes that by Tennant and Andrews (1976), who measured life change and distress; Dohrenwend et al. (1978), who developed the Psychiatric Epidemiology Research Interview Life Events Scale; and Paykel (1983), who in the late 1960s developed the Interview for Recent Life Events.

Another significant contribution to the measurement of recent life events was provided by George Brown and colleagues in the form of the Life Event and Difficulty Schedule (Brown and Harris 1978, 1989). This semistructured interview sought to reduce interjudge variability in rating stressors by eliciting information about the context in which events occurred. This context is constructed to take into account the meaning of events for a given individual based on his or her life circumstance, yet without including the individual's assessment of the magnitude of the event or information on the individual's personal reaction to the event. Standardized ratings are performed to evaluate a stressor in terms of the magnitude of stress that would be experienced by most persons in this type of situation.

This method of assessing a stressor in the form of a contextual threat has produced strong associations between life events and physical health outcomes. However, it has been argued that this method engenders the problem of basing ratings on variables that may be risk factors. For example, as Tennant et al. (1981) pointed out, contextual variables such as "employment status, the number of children at home, and the nature of the relationship with spouse or lover are used to define the degree of threat" (p. 380) for a particular stressor, yet these situational or personal variables may as likely account for the relationship to outcome as the event being assessed.

Despite this criticism, the issue of how to account for context remains unresolved. Thus, some researchers continue to favor the method of contextual assessment of events, whereas others continue to favor independent measurement of stressors. This latter group, however, adds the caveat that information must be elicited to understand an event thoroughly, thus reducing interjudge variability in assessing the normative value of event magnitude (Dohrenwend et al. 1993).

Continuing attention to the issue that events may have different meanings has also led, at least in part, to research that has begun to address a third major issue that arises in assessing life events: Certain types of stressors may have differential effects. In fact, certain types of stressors either result in different manifestations of illness or may affect patient groups differently. Some of the distinctions generated to categorize different types of stressors include 1) relatively acute events, such as a sudden death, versus a lingering chronic experience, such as long-standing marital conflict; 2) minor stressors, or "daily hassles" (Lazarus and Folkman 1984), versus major events, such as death of a loved one; 3) generally desirable events, such as birth of a child, versus undesirable events, which usually signify loss; and 4) events that might respond to one's control by making a life adjustment, such as leaving an unsatisfying job, versus those events relatively outside one's control, such as the experience of chronic pain following an accident.

In reference to the acute versus chronic differentiation, for example, Hammen et al. (1992) found that acute stressors interact differently than chronic stressors with other variables, such as age at onset or family history, to predict severity of depression. Others have also hypothesized that exposure to acute versus chronic stressors may result in different forms of illness. Specifically, chronic stressors may be associated with chronic forms of illness such as dysthymic disorder (Brown et al. 1986).

Adverse reactions to minor stressors have also been a focus of study, and some researchers have indicated that such reactions may be better indications of vulnerability to illness than reactions to major stressors. In a further clarification of the desirable/undesirable distinction, researchers such as Finlay-Jones and Brown (1981) and Paykel (1982) have suggested that major life events representing loss may predict onset of depression, whereas events that indicate danger may initiate episodes of anxiety disorders.

Uncontrollable stress may be particularly pernicious for certain groups, such as those suffering from posttraumatic stress disorder, or for depressed patients (Breier 1989). Or it may be the inability to accept the lack of control that turns uncomplicated bereavement into major depression (Jacobs 1992). Other types of stressors have also been hypothesized to be important dimensions of an event. For example, Dohrenwend et al. (1993), in addition to measuring undesirability and degree to which an event is under one's control, also measure if events are life threatening and if life change associated with an event is likely to be physically exhausting.

In sum, assessment of stressful life events has been a difficult issue for those wishing to pursue the relationship of stress and illness. Within the domain of life events, only a subset of such occurrences may be related to the onset of certain disorders in certain vulnerable individuals. This potentially intricate relationship between types of stressors and psychiatric illness is yet to be understood. However, advancements have been made to address the issues encountered in measuring stressors. These steps have allowed researchers to begin to generate empirical data that inform us about this complex and clinically relevant relationship.

CONCLUSION

We have attempted to present an overview of early conceptual models on the etiology of mental illness to examine the role of stressors in those theories. Our discussion of whether or how stressful life events fit into these models was limited by available primary historical information and the focus of secondary sources of information. However, we have discussed general trends in thinking while acknowledging that there are always exceptions to the rule. It seems that the evolution of knowledge about the etiology of mental illness, and the inclusion of external stressors in theoretical conceptualizations, are marked by fits and starts. It may progress and then seemingly stall or even temporarily reverse itself. However, in general, until relatively modern times, theories of mental illness did not focus on whether or how stressors, and particularly stressful life events, had a direct impact on the development of disorders. Modern nosology, as a reflection of contemporary theoretical positions, has seemingly embraced the notion that stressors relate to at least some disorders and has begun to search for the best way to characterize that relationship. However, just as the nosology continues to be revised, so too will the manner in which psychosocial stress is evaluated. Both biological and psychosocially based studies have provided a rich tradition with which to continue the investigation of this issue. The emphasis for the next generation of researchers appears to be found in increasing attempts to specify the disorders and concepts under study and integrating biological and psychosocial factors in understanding the complex relationship of stress and mental illness.

REFERENCES

Ackernecht EH: A Short History of Psychiatry. New York, Hafner Publishing, 1968

Akiskal HS: Is stress a predisposing or precipitating factor in clinical depression? Behavioral and Brain Sciences 5:99–100, 1982

Akiskal HS, McKinney WT Jr: Depressive disorders: toward a unified hypothesis. Science 182:20–29, 1973

Akiskal HS, McKinney WT Jr: Overview of recent research in depression: an integration of conceptual models into a comprehensive clinical frame. Arch Gen Psychiatry 32:285–301, 1975

Alexander FG, Selesnick ST: The History of Psychiatry. New York, Harper & Row, 1966

Ambelas A: Psychologically stressful events in the precipitation of manic episodes. Br J Psychiatry 135:15–21, 1979

Ambelas A: Life events and mania: a special relationship. Br J Psychiatry 150:235–240, 1987

American Psychiatric Association: Diagnostic and Statistical Manual: Mental Disorders. Washington, DC, American Psychiatric Association, 1952

American Psychiatric Association: Diagnostic and Statistical Manual of Mental Disorders, 2nd Edition. Washington, DC, American Psychiatric Association, 1968

American Psychiatric Association: Diagnostic and Statistical Manual of Mental Disorders, 3rd Edition. Washington, DC, American Psychiatric Association, 1980

American Psychiatric Association: Diagnostic and Statistical Manual of Mental Disorders, 3rd Edition, Revised. Washington, DC, American Psychiatric Association, 1987

American Psychiatric Association: Diagnostic and Statistical Manual of Mental Disorders, 4th Edition. Washington, DC, American Psychiatric Association, 1994

Aneshensel CS, Stone JD: Stress and depression: a test of the buffering model of social support. Arch Gen Psychiatry 39:1392–1396, 1982

Barnett PA, Gotlib IH: Psychosocial functioning and depression: distinguishing among antecedents, concomitants and consequences. Psychol Bull 104:97–126, 1988

Battie W: A Treatise on Madness (1758). New York, Brunner/Mazel, 1969

Bebbington PE, Brugha T, MacCarthy B, et al: The Camberwell Collaborative Depression Study; I: depressed probands: adversity and the form of depression. Br J Psychiatry 152:754–765, 1988

Berman KF, Torrey EF, Daniel DG, et al: Regional cerebral blood flow in monozygotic twins discordant for schizophrenia. Arch Gen Psychiatry 49:927–934, 1992

Bidzinska EJ: Stress factors in affective diseases. Br J Psychiatry 144:161–166, 1984

Birch PJ, Anderson SMP, Fillenz M: Mild chronic stress leads to desensitization of presynaptic autoreceptors and a long-lasting increase in noradrenaline synthesis in rat cortical synaptosomes. Neurochemistry International 9:329–336, 1986

Birley J, Brown GW: Crisis and life changes preceding the onset or relapse of acute schizophrenia: clinical aspects. Br J Psychiatry 16:327–333, 1970

Blashfield RK: The Classification of Psychopathology: Neo-Kraepelinian and Quantitative Approaches. New York, Plenum, 1984

Bowers MB Jr, Mazure CM, Nelson JC, et al: Psychotogenic drug use and neuroleptic response. Schizophr Bull 16:81–85, 1990

Breier A: Experimental approaches to human stress research: assessment of neurobiological mechanisms of stress in volunteers and psychiatric patients. Biol Psychiatry 26:438–462, 1989

Breier A, Kelsoe JR, Kirwin PD, et al: Early parental loss and development of adult psychopathology. Arch Gen Psychiatry 45:987–993, 1988

Brown GW, Birley JL: Crises and life changes and the onset of schizophrenia. J Health Soc Behav 9:203–214, 1968

Brown GW, Harris TO: Social Origins of Depression: A Study of Psychiatric Disorder in Women. New York, Free Press, 1978

Brown GW, Harris TO: Life Events and Illness. New York, Guilford, 1989

Brown GW, Bifulco A, Harris TO, et al: Life stress, chronic subclinical symptoms and vulnerability to clinical depression. J Affect Disord 11:1–19, 1986

Brown GW, Bifulco A, Harris TO: Life events, vulnerability and the onset of depression: some refinements. Br J Psychiatry 150:30–42, 1987

Burton R: The Anatomy of Melancholia (1621). New York, Tudor Publishing Company, (copyright by Farrar & Rinehart), 1927

Cassano GB, Akiskal HS, Musetti L, et al: Psychopathology, temperament, and past course in primary major depressions, II: toward a redefinition of bipolarity with a new semistructured interview for depression. Psychopathology 22:278–288, 1989

Chrousos GP, Gold PW: The concepts of stress and stress system disorders: overview of physical and behavioral homeostasis. JAMA 267:1244–1252, 1992

Cohen S, Wills TA: Stress, social support and the buffering hypothesis. Psychol Bull 98:310–357, 1985

Cooper B: Mental disorder as reaction: the history of a psychiatric concept, in Life Events and Psychiatric Disorders: Controversial Issues. Edited by Katschnig H. Cambridge, England, Cambridge University Press, 1986, pp 1–32

Day R, Nielson JA, Korten G, et al: Stressful life events preceding the acute onset of schizophrenia: a cross-national study from the World Health Organization. Cult Med Psychiatry 11:123–205, 1987

Deutch AY, Clark WA, Roth RH: Prefrontal cortical dopamine depletion enhances the responsiveness of mesolimbic dopamine neurons to stress. Brain Res 521:311–315, 1990

Dohrenwend BS, Krasnoff L, Askenasy AR, et al: Exemplification of a method for scaling life events: the PERI life events scale. J Health Soc Behav 19:205–229, 1978

Dohrenwend BP, Steuve A, Skodol AE: Life events and schizophrenia with some comparisons to major depression: a case/control study. Paper presented at the annual meeting of the American Psychiatric Association, Washington, DC, May 1992

Dohrenwend BP, Raphael KG, Schwarz S, et al: The structured event probe and narrative rating method (SEPRATE) for measuring stressful life events, in Handbook of Stress: Theoretical and Clinical Aspects, 2nd Edition. Edited by Goldberger L, Bresnitz S. New York, Free Press, 1993, pp 174–199

Dolan RJ, Calloway SP, Fonagy P, et al: Life events, depression, and hypothalamic-pituitary-adrenal axis function. Br J Psychiatry 147:429–433, 1985

Egeland JA, Gerhard DS, Pauls DL, et al: Bipolar affective disorders linked to DNA markers on chromosome 11. Nature 325:783–787, 1987

Ezquiaga E, Gutierrez JLA, Lopez AG: Psychosocial factors and episode number in depression. J Affect Disord 12:135–138, 1987

Finlay-Jones R, Brown GW: Types of stressful life events and the onset of anxiety and depressive disorders. Psychol Med 11:803–815, 1981

Flaherty JA, Gaviria FM, Black EM, et al: The role of social support in the functioning of patients with unipolar depression. Am J Psychiatry 140:473–476, 1983

Freud S: Mourning and melancholia (1917), in The Standard Edition of the Complete Psychological Works of Sigmund Freud, Vol 14. Translated and edited by Strachey J. London, Hogarth Press, 1957, pp 243–258

Freud S: Anxiety and instinctual life (1933), in New Introductory Lectures on Psychoanalysis: Sigmund Freud. Translated and edited by Strachey J. New York, WW Norton, 1965, pp 81–111

Ghaziuddin M, Ghaziuddin N, Stein GS: Life events and the recurrence of depression. Can J Psychiatry 35:239–242, 1990

Glavin G: Stress and brain noradrenaline: a review. Neuroscience Biobehavioral Review 9:233–243, 1985

Gold PW, Goodwin FK, Chrousos GP: Clinical and biochemical manifestations of depression: II. N Engl J Med 319:413–420, 1988

Goshen CE: Documentary History of Psychiatry: A Source Book on Historical Principles. New York, Philosophical Library, 1967

Gordon RE, Jardiolin P, Gordon KK: Predicting length of hospital stay of psychiatric patients. Am J Psychiatry 142:235–237, 1985

Griesinger W: Mental Pathology and Therapeutics (1867). Translated by Robertson CL, Rutherford J. New York, William Wood, 1882

Grob GN: Mental Institutions in America: Social Policy to 1875. New York, Free Press, 1973

Grove WM, Andreasen NC: Multivariate statistical analysis in psychopathology, in Contemporary Directions in Psychopathology: Toward the DSM-IV. Edited by Millon T, Klerman GL. New York, Guilford, 1986, pp 347–362

Guze SB, Cloninger CR, Martin RL, et al: A follow-up and family study of schizophrenia. Arch Gen Psychiatry 40:1273–1276, 1983

Haaga DAF, Dyck MJ, Ernst D: Empirical status of cognitive theory of depression. Psychol Bull 110:215–236, 1991

Hammen C: Generation of stress in the course of unipolar depression. J Abnorm Psychol 100:555–561, 1991

Hammen C, Ellicott A, Gitlin M, et al: Sociotropy/autonomy and vulnerability to specific life events in patients with unipolar depression and bipolar disorders. J Abnorm Psychol 98:154–160, 1989

Hammen C, Davila J, Brown G, et al: Psychiatric history and stress: predictors of severity of unipolar depression. J Abnorm Psychol 10:45–52, 1992

Holahan CJ, Moos RH: Life stressors, personal and social resources, and depression: a 4-year structural model. J Abnorm Psychol 100:31–38, 1991

Holmes TH, Rahe RH: The Social Readjustment Rating Scale. J Psychosom Res 11:213–218, 1967

Hunter R, Macalpine I: Three Hundred Years of Psychiatry. New York, Oxford University Press, 1963

Hyman SE, Nestler EJ: The Molecular Foundations of Psychiatry. Washington, DC, American Psychiatric Press, 1993

Jackson SW: Melancholia and Depression: From Hippocratic Times to Modern Times. New Haven, CT, Yale University Press, 1986

Jacobs S: Conscious and unconscious coping under stress, II: relationship to one and two years outcomes after bereavement. Paper presented at the annual meeting of the American Psychiatric Association, Washington, DC, May 1992

Katschnig H, Pakesch G, Egger-Zeidner E: Life stress and depressive subtypes: a review of present diagnostic criteria and recent research results, in Life Events and Psychiatric Disorders: Controversial Issues. Edited by Katschnig H. Cambridge, England, Cambridge University Press, 1986, pp 201–245

Kendler KS, Gruenberg AM, Tsuang MT: Psychiatric illness in first degree relatives of schizophrenic and surgical control patients: a family study using DSM-III criteria. Arch Gen Psychiatry 42:770–779, 1985

Kety SS: Mental illness in the biological and adoptive relatives of schizophrenic adoptees: findings relevant to genetic and environmental factors in etiology. Am J Psychiatry 140:720–727, 1983

Kraeplin E, Lange J: Psychiatrie, Neunte Auflage. Leipzig, Johann Ambrosius Barth, 1927

Lazarus RS, Folkman S: Stress, Appraisal and Coping. New York, Springer, 1984

Leff JP: A model of schizophrenic vulnerability to environmental factors, in Search for the Causes of Schizophrenia. Edited by Hafner H, Gattaz WF, Janzarik W. Berlin, Springer-Verlag, 1987, pp 317–330

Leff JP, Vaughn C: The interaction of life events and relatives expressed emotion in schizophrenia and depressive neurosis. Br J Psychiatry 136:146–153, 1980

Leff JP, Hirsch SR, Gaind R, et al: Life events and maintenance therapy in schizophrenic relapse. Br J Psychiatry 123:659–660, 1973

Lewinsohn PM, Hoberman HM, Rosenbaum M: A prospective study of risk factors for unipolar depression. J Abnorm Psychol 97:251–264 1988

Lloyd C, Zisook S, Click M, et al: Life events and response to antidepressants. J Human Stress 7:2–15, 1981

Lukoff D, Snyder K, Ventura J, et al: Life events, familial stress, and coping in the developmental course of schizophrenia. Schizophr Bull 12:258–292, 1984

Mason JW: A reevaluation of the concept of "non-specificity" in stress theory. J Psychiatry Res 8:323–333, 1971

Mason JW: A historical view of the stress field: I. Journal of Human Stress 1:6–12, 1975a

Mason JW: A historical view of the stress field: II. Journal of Human Stress 1:22–44, 1975b

McGue M, Gottesman II, Rao DC: The transmission of schizophrenia under a multifactorial threshold model. Am J Hum Genet 35:1161–1178, 1983

Meehl PE: Schizotaxia, schizotypy, schizophrenia. Am Psychol 17:827–838, 1962

Mendlewicz J, Rainer JD: Adoption study supporting genetic transmission in manic-depressive illness. Nature 268:327–329, 1977

Menninger K: The Vital Balance: The Life Process in Mental Health and Illness. New York, Viking Press, 1963

Mezzich JE, Evanczuk KJ, Mathias RJ, et al: Admission decisions and multiaxial diagnosis. Arch Gen Psychiatry 41:1001–1004, 1984

Miller P, Ingham NB, Kreitman PG, et al: Life events and other factors implicated in onset and remission of psychiatric illness in women. J Affect Disord 12:73–88, 1987

Millon T: On the past and future of the DSM-III: personal recollections and projections, in Contemporary Directions in Psychopathology: Toward the DSM-IV. Edited by Millon T, Klerman GL. New York, Guilford, 1986, pp 29–70

Monroe SM, Depue RA: Life stress and depression, in Psychosocial Aspects of Depression. Edited by Becker J, Kleinman A. Hillside, NJ, Erlbaum, 1991, pp 101–130

Monroe SM, Simons AD: Diathesis/stress theories in the context of life stress research: implications for the depressive disorders. Psychol Bull 110:406–425, 1991

Monroe SM, Bellack AS, Hersen M, et al: Life events, symptom course and treatment outcome in unipolar depressed women. J Consult Clin Psychol 51:604–615, 1983

Oxford English Dictionary: Second Edition. Prepared by Simpson JA. Oxford, England, Clarendon Press, 1989

Packan DR, Sapolsky RM: Glucocorticoid endangerment of the hippo-campus: tissue, steroid and receptor specificity. Neuroendocrinology 51:613–618, 1990

Paykel ES: Recent life events in the development of the depressive disorders, in The Psychobiology of the Depressive Disorders: Implications for the Effects of Stress. Edited by Depue RA. New York, Academic Press, 1979, pp 245–262

Paykel ES: Life events and early environment, in Handbook of Affective Disorders. Edited by Paykel ES. New York, Guilford, 1982, pp 146–161

Paykel ES: Methodological aspects of life event research. J Psychosom Res 27:341–352, 1983

Paykel ES, Tanner J: Life events, depressive relapse and maintenance treatment. Psychol Med 6:481–485, 1976

Pearlin LI, Schooler C: The structure of coping. J Health Soc Behav 19:2–21, 1978

Perris H: Life events and depression, II: results in diagnostic subgroups and in relation to the recurrence of depression. J Affect Disord 7:25–36, 1984

Post RM: Transduction of psychosocial stress into the neurobiology of recurrent affective disorder. Am J Psychiatry 149:999–1010, 1992

Rosen G: Social stress and mental disease from the eighteenth century to the present: some origins of social psychiatry. Milbank Memorial Fund Quarterly 37:5–32, 1959

Rutter M: Resilience in the face of adversity: protective factors and resistance to psychiatric disorder. Br J Psychiatry 147:598–611, 1985

Schrader G, Gordon M, Harcourt R: The usefulness of DSM-III Axis IV and Axis V assessments. Am J Psychiatry 143:904–907, 1986

Segal ZV, Shaw BF, Vella DD, et al: Cognitive and life stress predictors of relapse in remitted unipolar depressed patients: test of the congruency hypothesis. J Abnorm Psychol 101:26–36, 1992

Selye H: A syndrome produced by diverse nocuous agents. Nature 138:32, 1936

Selye H: The Stress of Life. New York, McGraw-Hill, 1956

Shrout PE, Link BG, Dohrenwend BP, et al: Characterizing life events as risk factors for depression: the role of fateful loss events. J Abnorm Psychol 984:460–467, 1989

Skodol AE, Shrout PE: Use of DSM-III Axis IV in clinical practice: rating the severity of psychological stressors. Psychiatry Res 30:201–211, 1989

Spring B, Coons H: Stress as a precursor of schizophrenia, in Psychological Stress and Psychopathology. Edited by Neufeld RWJ. New York, McGraw-Hill, 1982, pp 13–54

Swindle R, Cronkite RC, Moos RH: Life stressors, social resources, coping and the 4-year course of unipolar depression. J Abnorm Psychol 98:468–477, 1989

Tennant C, Andrews G: A scale to measure the stress of life events. Aust N Z J Psychiatry 10:27–32, 1976

Tennant C, Bebbington P, Hurry J: The role of life events in depressive illness: is there a substantial causal relation? Psychol Med 11:379–389, 1981

Torgerson S: Genetic factors in anxiety disorders. Arch Gen Psychiatry 40:1085–1089, 1983

Tsuang MT, Winokur G, Crowe RR: Morbidity risks of schizophrenia and affective disorders among first degree relatives of patients with schizophrenia, mania, depression, and surgical conditions. Br J Psychiatry 137:497–504, 1980

Turpin G, Lader M: Life events and mental disorder: biological theories of their mode of action, in Life Events and Psychiatric Disorders: Controversial Issues. Edited by Katschnig H. Cambridge, England, Cambridge University Press, 1986, pp 33–62

Ventura J, Nuechterlein KH, Hardesty JP, et al: Life events and schizophrenic relapse after medication withdrawal. Br J Psychiatry 161:615–620, 1992

Vingerhoets A: Psychosocial Stress: An Experimental Approach. Lisse, The Netherlands, Swets & Zeitlinger, 1985

Weinberger DR, Berman KF, Suddath R, et al: Evidence of dysfunction of a prefrontal-limbic network in schizophrenia: a magnetic resonance imaging and regional cerebral blood flow study of discordant monozygotic twins. Am J Psychiatry 149:890–897, 1992

Weiner DB: Philippe Pinel's "Memoir on Madness" of December 11, 1794: a fundamental text of modern psychiatry. Am J Psychiatry 149:725–732, 1992

Weiss JM, Stone EA, Harrell N: Coping behavior and brain norepinephrine level in rats. Journal of Comparative and Physiological Psychology 72:153–160, 1970

Wender PH, Kety SS, Rosenthal D, et al: Psychiatric disorders in the biological and adoptive families of adopted individuals with affective disorders. Arch Gen Psychiatry 43:923–929, 1986

Williams JBW: The multiaxial system of DSM-III: where did it come from and where should it go? I: its origins and critiques. Arch Gen Psychiatry 42:175–180, 1985

World Health Organization: International Classification of Diseases, 8th Edition. Geneva, Switzerland, World Health Organization, 1968

World Health Organization: International Classification of Diseases, 9th Edition. Geneva, Switzerland, World Health Organization, 1979

Zimmerman M, Pfohl B, Stangl D, et al: The validity of DSM-III Axis IV (severity of psychosocial stressors). Am J Psychiatry 142:1437–1441, 1985

Zimmerman M, Pfohl B, Coryell W, et al: The prognostic validity of DSM-III Axis IV in depressed inpatients. Am J Psychiatry 144:102–106, 1987

Zubin J, Spring B: Vulnerability: a new view of schizophrenia. J Abnorm Psychol 86:103–126, 1977

Chapter 2

Life Events and Other Possible Psychosocial Risk Factors for Episodes of Schizophrenia and Major Depression: A Case-Control Study

Bruce P. Dohrenwend, Ph.D.,
Patrick E. Shrout, Ph.D.,
Bruce G. Link, Ph.D.,
Andrew E. Skodol, M.D.,
and Ann Stueve, Ph.D.

I t has long been evident that a variety of social circumstances and personal characteristics are likely to affect the impact of stressful life events on a person's health (e.g., B. S. Dohrenwend and Dohrenwend 1974, 1981a; Rabkin and Struening 1976). This recognition has been slow, however, to influence research on relations between life events and major psychiatric disorders such as schizophrenia and depression.

Lukoff et al. (1984) pointed out, for example, that the relevant

This study was supported by U.S. Public Health Service Grants MH36208, K5-MH14663, MH38773, T32-MH13034, MH30906; National Science Foundation Grant DAR-80-08463; and a grant from the National Alliance for Research on Schizophrenia and Depression. We thank the following people for their help in this chapter: Matthias C. Angermeyer, M.D., Michael Flory, Ph.D., Miriam Gibbon, M.S.W, Ewald Horvath, M.D., Rochelle Kern, Ph.D., Mary Clare Lennon, Ph.D., Jerrold Mirotznick, Ph.D., Karen Raphael, Ph.D., Robert Spitzer, M.D., and Janet Williams, D.S.W.

research on life events and schizophrenia tended to be limited to investigations using "a two variable design" concentrated exclusively on assessing the occurrence of life events prior to the occurrence of a schizophrenic episode. A more recent review by Norman and Malla (1993) indicated that there has been little change in this narrow approach. The focus is beginning to be expanded in research on life events and depression. Although none of the studies include a great variety of other psychosocial variables, such social factors as the presence of a confidant and the number of young children in the home have been included in the case-control study of life events and depression by Brown and Harris (1978), depression-related cognitions were investigated in a prospective study by Lewinsohn et al. (1988), and family history of disorder was included in research by Hammen et al. (1992) and McGuffin et al. (1987).

In the present study, we attempted to include a much larger number and greater variety of stress-related social, psychological, and family history variables than have been previously investigated together in relation to episodes of schizophrenia or schizophrenia-like disorders and episodes of major depression. These possible risk factors were selected on the basis of previous research and theory about relations between stress and adverse health changes (B. S. Dohrenwend and Dohrenwend 1981). They are organized within the framework of our conceptualization of life stress processes (B. S. Dohrenwend and Dohrenwend 1981; B. P. Dohrenwend et al. 1993), which are seen as consisting of three main components.

The first component is recent events that may occur within a relatively brief time interval (usually a few months to a year) prior to an episode of disorder. These events can range from extreme situations, such as prolonged exposure to combat during wartime or a natural disaster, to more usual life events, such as the birth of a child, the death of a loved one, getting a new job, losing a job, and so on.

The second component is the ongoing situation. This consists of various long-standing circumstances that may have current impact. Major facets of the ongoing situation include domestic arrangements with regard to child care and housekeeping and the types of occupations in which an individual is employed. In addition, there is the role of social networks consisting of family, friends, and acquaintances who are potential sources of social support.

The third component comprises the personal dispositions of the individual. Under personal dispositions we include vulnerabilities related to family history of mental disorder and the possibly adverse effects on present personality of remote events such as early childhood bereavement. We include also the experience of past disorder. We consider as well a set of personality characteristics that are distinct from psychopathology but that are likely to contribute to how the individual copes with stress.

In this chapter we first summarize which variables in each of these three components of life stress processes differentiate known cases of each type of disorder from each other and from control subjects who suffer from neither type of disorder. Next, we discuss the limitations of this first step in identifying firm risk factors. Finally, we outline the steps we are taking to test these possible risk factors further as we attempt to understand their interrelationships and to assess their implications for etiology, treatment, and prevention.

METHOD

The data come from 65 patients who experienced recent episodes of nonaffective functional psychotic disorders: 21 first-episode and 44 repeat-episode cases. The majority (30 of 44) of the repeat-episode cases met DSM-III (American Psychiatric Association 1980) criteria for schizophrenia, with the remainder consisting of schizoaffective, paranoid, schizophreniform, and atypical psychoses. These 65 cases of nonaffective psychotic disorder were compared with 96 cases of major depression (49 first episode) and 404 control subjects sampled from the general population. The control subjects were screened to remove persons meeting criteria for current major depression and nonaffective functional psychotic disorder. The diagnoses by psychiatric residents were systematically reviewed by members of the Biometrics Research Department of the New York State Psychiatric Institute according to procedures described by Skodol et al. (1984). Additional details of sampling and completion rates are provided elsewhere (Link et al. 1989; Shrout et al. 1989).

Recent Life Events

The patients were interviewed about life events in the year prior to the episode for which they were selected and the control subjects for the year prior to the interview. The respondents were asked first about the occurrence of both positive and negative events on a checklist containing 88 content categories plus a category for "other" events that might not have been included (B. S. Dohrenwend et al. 1982). Reports of negative events were probed by the interviewers with questions about when they occurred and what actually happened and about changes in usual activities following the events.

On the basis of this narrative information from respondents, a variety of ratings were made by the research team about objective aspects of the events that were thought to be important in determining the nature of their impact. One of the most important of these ratings focuses on the extent to which the respondent's behavior, rather than external circumstances, affected the sequence leading up to the event and the event's actual occurrence. (For example, for an event involving being fired from a job, the prelude might involve being late to work and doing a poor job; the immediate act would involve dismissal by the boss.) In addition, an overall judgment was made of the likelihood that personal dispositions influenced the occurrence of the event. These ratings are crucial in assessing the extent to which a negative event was "fateful"—that is, the extent to which its occurrence is an indicator of environmental adversity (B. P. Dohrenwend 1979; B. P. Dohrenwend et al. 1993).

The amount of change in usual activities following the event was also evaluated to provide a measure of magnitude. For fateful events, the rating was for the amount of change in usual activities the average person to whom the event occurred would be likely to experience. This type of normative rating was adopted to avoid confounding the assessment of the objective magnitude with differences in coping ability that would be likely to affect the amount of change reported by different individuals in relation to the same event. For nonfateful events, where personal dispositions that were likely to affect coping play a part in the occurrence of the event, the need to secure normative ratings of change was thought to be less important; therefore, the ratings used were made of the actual amount of change taking place for the particular person who experienced the event. For physical illness and injury events, we substituted ratings of seriousness by physicians for the change ratings as the measure of magnitude; the physicians used the rating procedures and examples of Wyler et al. (1968) as guides for their judgments.

These ratings enabled us to classify negative events not only as fateful versus nonfateful but also as "major" (involving more than moderate change), "moderate," and "minor" (involving little change likely to last a week or more or no change likely to last a week or more). Since most of the negative events were dated to month of occurrence, it was possible to focus on the period of 3 months prior to episode (for patients) or interview (for control subjects) for purposes of comparability to other research, especially the classic study of schizophrenic episodes conducted by Brown and Birley (1968). More details of the rationale for this approach to measuring life events and its further development are provided elsewhere (B. P. Dohrenwend et al. 1993).

Ongoing Social Situation

We inquired into three main aspects of the ongoing situation prior to the onset of disorder that were more remote in origin than the recent life events: 1) the personal network of the respondent, including the existence of a close confidant; 2) characteristics of his or her occupation that might be stressful; and, especially for women; 3) domestic arrangements related to child care, care of home, and the business of shopping, providing meals, and so on (Brown and Harris 1978; Pearlin and Johnson 1977).

We followed the procedure developed by Fischer (1982) for eliciting the members of the personal networks of our cases and control subjects. Briefly, this involved asking each respondent to name those individuals with whom he or she had, or could have had, supportive exchanges in the following areas of activity: care of children, watching the house while he or she was away, discussion of decisions at work, discussion of personal problems, borrowing money, and social and recreational activities. From this information, we constructed such social support network variables as size and extensiveness (the number of areas covered and the depth of coverage).

We developed two measures of whether and to what extent the respondent had a close confidant. The first was constructed to approximate Brown and Harris's (1978) definition of confidant intimacy. Respondents were rated as having a high intimacy relationship if at least one household member (the spouse for married couples) was someone with whom the respondent discussed worries or whose advice the respondent considered in decision making.

Second, to examine the process through which the confiding relationship functions as a form of social support, self-disclosure to the respondent's closest network member was evaluated. Respondents completed a modified form (Raphael and Dohrenwend 1987) of the Jourard Self-Disclosure Questionnaire (JSDQ; Jourard 1971). The JSDQ evaluated a respondent's self-disclosure to the network member with whom he or she felt closest by asking how much that network member knew about the respondent based on a list of personal topics. Topics related to disclosure of body image, personality, interests, attitudes, and personal history were included. The 21-item form that we used has internal consistency reliabilities better than .80 in each case and control group.

Domestic arrangements included, in addition to marital status, which was statistically controlled in all these analyses, the variables of child care responsibility and housework burden. Child care responsibility was measured with three categories, ranging from low to high: 1) no children under age 14 in the home; 2) children under 14 at home and some help with child care; and 3) children under 14 and no child care help. The "under 14" cutoff point was based on findings by Brown and Harris (1978). Housework burden was also assessed using three ordinal levels: 1) no responsibility for housework; 2) some, but not entire, responsibility for housework; and 3) sole responsibility for housework.

Measures of occupational factors were constructed using the

Dictionary of Occupational Titles (DOT; U. S. Department of Labor 1977), which provides 44 ratings of the characteristics of 12,044 occupations (Cain and Treiman 1981). The ratings were made by U.S. Department of Labor analysts in on-site investigations of selected workplace locations. By coding the respondent's occupation at, or last occupation prior to, psychotic or depressive episode (for patients) and at, or prior to, interview (for control subjects) to the 9-digit DOT occupational codes, we were able to incorporate the 44 occupational conditions that are likely to be stressful. These include physical demands ($\alpha = .71$) and noisome work conditions involving hazards, noise, excessive humidity, and temperature extremes ($\alpha = .69$) (Link et al. 1986). We also used a DOT rating that we did not include in these composite measures, that of repetitive and continuous tasks.

Personal Dispositions

We constructed or adapted measures of two sets of dispositional factors: a set of normal personality variables and a set of various remote events and situations that might be expected to have affected the current personality of the individual. Under the latter set, we included presence of a family history of mental disorder.

Our choice of personality measures included the scales of locus of control developed by Rotter (1966) and Levenson (1972), Jenkins et al.'s (1967) measure of Type A behavior, a set of items that we are calling "mastery orientation" from the Spence and Helmreich (1978) measures of masculinity and femininity, a set of items that seem to indicate passive emotionality from the same source, and two scales developed by Miller (1980) to identify individuals who are likely to monitor stress situations closely for details of what is taking place by contrast with individuals who tend to blunt or deny what is going on. We tested the internal consistency reliabilities of these measures, and they were satisfactory, ranging from about .80 to .60 for the various scales among all the respondents combined and never less than .50 in either case group or the control subjects.

We included questions on the following remote events and situations: death of mother or father during childhood, being raised by someone other than mother or father, whether the respondents or their friends were in trouble with authorities before age 18, past life-threatening physical illnesses and injuries, and family history of mental disorders. The last two of these require further description.

We asked the respondents to list the three most serious physical illnesses and/or injuries they had ever had. They were also asked to say when each of the illnesses or injuries occurred, whether it still bothered them, and whether it was life threatening. We also administered a checklist of specific past illnesses that were scored for seriousness of illness (Wyler et al. 1968).

Our measure of family history was primitive. We used reports by the respondents about the psychiatric problems of their first-degree relatives rather than the more satisfactory procedure of conducting direct interviews with the relatives themselves (Orvaschel et al. 1982). We also did not question in detail about symptomatology. Each respondent was asked whether each of his or her first-degree relatives had ever had "serious mental or emotional problems such as problems with depression, suicide attempts, odd or violent behavior, or difficulties with drugs or alcohol." If the answer was affirmative, the respondent was further asked to name "the specific mental or emotional problem(s) that the relative(s) had" and whether the relative was "ever in a hospital" for the specific problem. If outpatient treatment was mentioned, this was recorded. Two psychiatrists independently rated the replies for evidence of the presence of disorder, achieving a kappa of .71, indicating satisfactory reliability (B. P. Dohrenwend et al. 1986).

STATISTICAL PROCEDURES

The analyses that we summarize involved comparisons of the two case groups with each other and with the well control subjects on the candidate social and psychological risk factor variables. Our statistical procedure was to test differences among the case and control groups after statistically controlling demographic factors that could affect these differences.

In all comparisons, the following variables were controlled:

sex, ethnicity (black, Hispanic, other), education (less than high school, high school graduate, college graduate), marital status (never married, divorced or separated, married), age (as a continuous variable), the respondent's father's occupational prestige (also continuous), and interaction between ethnicity and father's occupational prestige.

For risk factors represented by quantitative variables, the statistical method used to adjust for demographic differences was the general linear model with least-squares estimation. In applying this method, we specified the risk factor as the dependent variable in a model containing the control variables as predictors and then tested the increase in fit resulting from the inclusion of indicators of diagnostic group. For categorical risk factors, an analogous procedure was used, with maximum likelihood logistic regression providing the statistical method.

Table 2–1 summarizes the variables investigated in each of the domains of recent life events, ongoing situation, and personal dispositions. Within each of the three domains of potential risk factors, we examined a wide variety of the specific variables for associations with the diagnostic group. Each association was further examined by considering three possible contrasts between pairs of the case and control groups. Clearly the overall probability of one or more Type I errors across all of these tests is larger than the nominal alpha used for each. However, to control the overall Type I error rate rigorously in all these tests would increase the probability of Type II error to such a level as to render our exploratory analyses meaningless. This is an especially severe problem with the smaller case group ($n = 65$) of individuals with schizophrenic episodes. With them, our power to detect differences from control subjects is less than with the larger group of 96 persons with major depressive episodes. Power is least of all for comparisons of each case group with the other.

To face these issues, we adopted the following policy in summarizing the results in Tables 2–2, 2–3, and 2–4 for the variables listed in Table 2–1. First, we present alpha levels for each specific comparison of a case group with the control group or with the other case group without adjusting for multiple tests. Second, within each risk factor domain (i.e., recent life events, ongoing situation, personal dispositions), we calculate the probability

Table 2–1. Summary of possible risk factors in three domains: recent life events, ongoing social situation, and personal dispositions

Recent life events (6 variables)	Ongoing social situation (10 variables)	Personal dispositions (22 variables)
Negative events in 3 months prior to episode (cases) or interview (control subjects): Major fateful Moderate fateful Minor fateful Major nonfateful Moderate nonfateful Minor nonfateful	Networks: Size Extensiveness Instrumental supporters Confiding relationships: Intimate confidant Self-disclosure to intimate confidant Domestic arrangements: Child care burden Housework burden Occupational characteristics: Noisome (e.g., excessive heat, cold, noise) Repetitiveness Physical arduousness	Personality variables: Locus of control (Rotter, Levenson) Type A Mastery orientation Blunters Monitors Passive emotionality Remote events or situations: Death of mother before respondent was 11 Separation from parents for a year or more before age 18 Mother as household head Raised by mother with no knowledge of father Raised in institution Friends in trouble with law enforcement authorities before age 18 Respondent in trouble with law enforcement authorities before age 18 Death of one or more of respondent's children

Past life-threatening illness or injury
Seriousness of past illness

Family history of disorder in one or more
  first-degree relatives:
  One or more first-degree relatives with
    probable mental disorder
  One or more first-degree relatives with
    each of the following subtypes
    Affective
    Psychotic
    Antisocial
    Alcoholism

level needed to satisfy the Bonferroni rule for an overall .05 Type I error rate, and we indicate with an asterisk which risk factor associations meet this criterion. These asterisked results are the associations that we are most confident will replicate.

RESULTS

Recent Life Events

The first set of results is on recent life events (Table 2–2). Fateful events, it will be recalled, are negative events for which occurrence was rated as outside the respondent's control and independent of his or her personality characteristics and behaviors. Respondents who had episodes of major depression were most likely to have experienced one or more antecedent major events on this measure, differing from both those who developed nonaffective psychotic episodes and the control subjects. Moderate and minor fateful events were not elevated in the cases of major depression compared with the other two groups. There is no significant elevation of fateful events (major, moderate, or minor) for persons with nonaffective psychotic disorders.

The picture is somewhat different for nonfateful negative

Table 2–2.   Recent negative life events measures that differentiated between each case group and control subjects and/or between case groups at .05 level with (*) and without a Bonferroni correction

Type of case	More at risk than control subjects	More at risk than other case group
Nonaffective functional psychotic disorders	One or more combined major, moderate, and minor nonfateful events	
Major depression	One or more major fateful events*	Major fateful*
	One or more major nonfateful events*	

events. Major nonfateful events, like major fateful events, differentiate major depressive cases from control subjects. However, unlike fateful events, nonfateful events may also play a part in the occurrence of nonaffective psychotic episodes.

Respondents with episodes of nonaffective psychotic disorders were more likely than control subjects to have reported nonfateful negative events. However, this occurred only when major, moderate, and minor events were combined, and even then the difference barely achieved statistical significance at the .05 level without a Bonferroni correction for multiple comparisons.

Ongoing Situation

Personal networks. The results summarized in Table 2–3 indicate that the networks of the respondents with nonaffective

Table 2–3. Measures of the ongoing situation that differentiated between each case group and control subjects and/or between case groups at .05 level with (*) and without Bonferroni correction

Type of case	More at risk than control subjects	More at risk than other case group
Nonaffective functional psychotic disorders	Network size*	Network size
	Network extensiveness*	Network extensiveness
	Instrumental supporters*	Instrumental supporters
	Intimate confidant	
	Noisome occupational characteristics	
Major depression	Network size	Housework burden*
	Network extensiveness*	
	Intimate confidant	
	Self-disclosure to intimate confidant	

psychotic episodes were the smallest and least extensive and had the fewest instrumental supporters compared with not only the control subjects but also with the cases of major depression. Although relatively strong compared with the respondents with cases of nonaffective psychoses, networks of the individuals with depressive episodes appear weak relative to the control subjects.

Confiding relationship. Both individuals with depressive episodes and those with episodes of nonaffective psychotic disorder were much less likely than well control subjects to report having an intimate relationship with a confidant. Since marital status is highly correlated with confidant intimacy, we repeated the analysis for married respondents only. The differences were even sharper.

Moreover, cases of both types appear less likely than control subjects to confide in the persons they described as closest to them. Self-disclosure (JSDQ) scores were lower for individuals with depressive episodes than for control subjects. There was a tendency for individuals who developed nonaffective psychotic episodes also to have lower JSDQ scores than control subjects, but, possibly because of the smaller n, the difference was not statistically significant at the .05 level ($P = .07$).

Domestic arrangements. Individuals who developed nonaffective psychotic episodes tended to have had less housework burden than either the depressive patients or control subjects; this tendency may be due to the dependent status of many of these cases. There appeared to be no differences in child care responsibility when relevant demographic variables were controlled. We looked specifically at whether there were differences in proportions with three or more children under age 14 living in the home. There were not, for females or males.

Occupational characteristics. Three occupational characteristics that we thought likely to be particularly stressful were tested: noisome characteristics, physical arduousness, and repetitiveness. There were no statistically significant differences in physical arduousness and repetitiveness. For respondents with nonaffective psychotic episodes, however, the occupation at the time of onset, or the last occupation before time of onset for those unemployed, tended to be characterized by noisome features such as excessive noise and temperature extremes. Moreover, as we reported previously, respondents with nonaffective psychotic episodes were substantially more likely to have engaged in first occupations with these characteristics after completing formal education than either patients with major depression or control subjects (Link et al. 1986).

Personal Dispositions

Personality variables. Table 2–4 summarizes comparisons on the personality variables. Note that, in contrast to the control subjects, respondents in both case groups tended to be high on external locus of control and low on mastery orientation. Thus, insofar as personality characteristics likely to be related to coping ability are concerned, both case groups were disadvantaged. Moreover, there were some differences between the two case groups. Compared both with respondents with nonaffective psychotic episodes and control subjects, individuals who developed depressive episodes endorsed more items indicating passive emotionality and Type A behavior. By contrast, respondents who developed episodes of nonaffective psychotic disorders were less likely to show monitoring responses than both control subjects and persons with depressive episodes. They were also more likely than control subjects to show blunter responses.

Remote events and situations. We have inquired into a number of past events and situations in the lives of our respondents. These results are also summarized in Table 2–4. Compared with control subjects, respondents in both case groups showed greater tendencies to report having had both friends who got into trouble with authorities before they were age 18 and more serious and more life-threatening past illnesses and injuries. In addition, respondents who developed episodes of nonaffective psychotic disorder were more likely than control subjects to report being raised by the mother alone and to have no knowledge of the father.

Family history. The case groups were found to differ in family history from the control subjects (Table 2–4). Both case groups were more likely to report at least one first-degree relative with a

Table 2–4. Measures of personal dispositions that differentiated between each case group and control subjects and/or between case groups at .05 level with (*) and without Bonferroni correction

Type of case	More at risk than control subjects	More at risk than other case group

Nonaffective functional psychotic disorders	Locus of control (Levenson)*
	Locus of control (Rotter)
	Mastery*
	Blunter
	Monitor
	Friends in trouble with authorities before age 18
	Past life-threatening illness or injury
	Seriousness of past illness or injury
	One or more first-degree relatives
	  with probable mental disorder*
	  with probable psychotic disorder
	  with probable alcoholism
		Monitors

Major depression	Locus of control (Levenson)*
	Locus of control (Rotter)
	Type A*
	Mastery*
	Passive emotionality*
	Raised mainly by mother with no knowledge of father
	Friends in trouble with authorities before age 18
	Past life-threatening illness or injury
	Seriousness of past illness or injury
	One or more first-degree relatives
	  with probable mental disorder*
	  with probable affective disorder*
	  with probable alcoholism
	  with probable antisocial behavior
		Type A
		Passive emotionality

probable mental disorder. Both case groups also tended to report more alcoholism among their first-degree relatives. There were also tendencies for individuals who developed episodes of non-affective psychotic disorder to report the highest rate of psychotic problems in their first-degree relatives, whereas persons who developed depressive episodes tended to report the highest rate of affective disorder.

DISCUSSION

We must reiterate that our analyses were designed to examine a multitude of risk factors with limited control for Type I error. The purpose of these analyses was to select variables that would be most likely to reward further investigation rather than provide decisive findings at this point. It is gratifying that, in this early stage of the analysis, a substantial number of the variables showed statistically significant differences among cases and control subjects even with a correction for multiple tests. Moreover, a number of the results are particularly worthy of attention because they bear on previous findings or appear to fit into a theoretical context. We believe such results not only are intrinsically more interesting but also are more likely to be ones that will replicate in future studies. We emphasize them in this discussion.

The findings indicate that recent life events do indeed play a larger role in episodes of depression than in episodes of schizophrenic disorder, as others have suggested (e.g., Brown and Harris 1978; Paykel 1974). Especially important is the fact that respondents with major depressive episodes were far more likely than individuals with nonaffective psychotic episodes to have experienced one or more major fateful events in the 90 days prior to the episode. Those fateful events were likely to be independent of personal dispositions and hence evidence of a role for recent environmentally induced stress. Not only were major fateful events elevated for individuals with episodes of depression, these events were also experienced by persons with stronger networks than had been available to individuals who developed episodes of nonaffective psychotic disorders.

It is harder to interpret the differences on personality variables. Along with the high external locus of control and low mastery orientations characteristic of both case groups, the individuals with depressive episodes gave more Type A and monitoring responses than individuals who developed nonaffective psychotic episodes. Given the retrospective nature of case-control studies, it is difficult to know whether the observed differences in personality predated illness onset or rather are consequences of psychopathology.

Although less than for major depression, there may be some role for recent events prior to episodes of nonaffective psychotic disorders. If so, however, it involves less severe events whose occurrence is more likely to be affected by personal dispositions and behavior. These patients appear to have not only weaker networks but also, possibly, more vulnerable personalities than the patients who developed episodes of depression or the control subjects. Note, for example, the elevated rate of blunting responses and the lower rate of monitoring response compared with the cases of major depression. It is possible that these personality differences are part of the reason that expressed negative emotions by the relatives toward discharged patients with schizophrenic disorders have been found to contribute to relapse (Leff and Vaughn 1981). Strong tendencies to blunt would be difficult to maintain in close family situations with highly critical relatives.

Recent stressful life events are not the only sources of environmental adversity that may be contributing to onset and recurrence of episodes of depression and episodes of nonaffective psychotic disorder. Both schizophrenia and major depression (at least in women) tend to be inversely related to socioeconomic status (Dohrenwend et al. 1992). This is especially evident in the present case samples. Some of our results indicate that individuals in our case samples tended to be exposed to adverse correlates of lower class circumstances occurring both early in life and in the ongoing situation prior to their episodes of disorder. Like the individuals with depressive episodes, those who developed episodes of nonaffective psychotic disorder tended to have had more stormy early environments, with families who had an excess of mental disorder and with their own life-threatening physical illnesses and injuries. For cases of nonaffective psychotic disorder, employment in occupations with noisome characteristics may constitute a particularly stressful transition from completion of formal education to beginning an occupational career (Link et al. 1986). We have argued elsewhere that exposure to such occupations is more likely to be a function of blue-collar family origins than a function of selection on the basis of personal dispositions specific to persons who develop schizophrenic episodes (Link et al. 1986). If so, these results on noisome occupations would be directly analogous to the World War II finding of unusually high rates of schizophrenic breakdown during the transition of inductees from civilian life into basic training (Steinberg and Durell 1968).

FUTURE STUDIES

We have planned two sets of further analyses to test, revise, and/or expand these interpretations. The first will focus on intensive analyses of variables within each of the three sets of potential risk factors: recent life events variables, factors in the ongoing situation, and variables measuring various aspects of personal dispositions. These investigations will include further tests of how firm each of the variables is as a risk factor. For example, we will check patient reporting of physical illnesses and injuries by reviewing their case records, and we will test how sensitive life event measures are to recall bias (e.g., Cohen et al. 1988; Raphael 1987). In addition, we plan to conduct analyses designed to investigate how likely the differences between cases and control subjects on personality variables and network variables are to be state-dependent functions of episodes of disorder for which the cases were selected (Hirschfeld et al. 1983). These investigations will include data from follow-up interviews with study subjects, some of whom were in episode-free periods, and analyses of the relation of these variables to demographic factors in the community sample.

In the second set of future analyses, we will examine the relation of recent life events to vulnerability (e.g., Zubin and Spring 1977). The first group of likely indicators of vulnerability will include whether the cases of nonaffective psychotic disorders and major depression were in their first-ever episode or in a repeat episode. We expect that, other things being equal, the first-episode cases will be a less vulnerable group. The type of episode onset (acute versus insidious) and the type of diagnosis (e.g., DSM-III schizophrenia versus other types of nonaffective psychotic disorders such as schizophreniform) should also be associated with greater or lesser vulnerability. Additional indicators of vulnerability will be chosen from the firmest and least redundant set of variables contained in Table 2–3 and Table 2–4. We will be especially interested, for example, in family history of various types of disorder as possible indicators of vulnerability and in those personality variables that prove not to be state dependent.

CONCLUSION

Several of the findings from the completed analyses summarized in Tables 2–2, 2–3, and 2–4 are too theoretically relevant, too strong, and/or too consistent with the other research not to be taken seriously, even now. Especially important theoretically, we think, are the results on the role of major fateful events in depression and the role of occupations with noisome characteristics in episodes of nonaffective psychotic disorders. These findings suggest that adverse environmental factors are indeed important in putting people at risk for episodes of depression (major fateful events) and episodes of nonaffective psychotic disorders (exposure to noisome occupational conditions). In addition, we must single out the results on psychiatric disorder in the first-degree relatives of persons with each type of disorder compared with the control subjects. Consistent with previous research on family history, the present results suggest that familial vulnerabilities loom large, be these transmitted genetically, through socialization processes, or both.

REFERENCES

American Psychiatric Association: Diagnostic and Statistical Manual of Mental Disorders, 3rd Edition. American Psychiatric Association, Washington, DC, 1980

Brown GW, Birley JLT: Crises and life changes and the onset of schizo-phrenia. J Health Soc Behav 9:203–214, 1968

Brown GW, Harris T: Social Origins of Depression. New York, Free Press, 1978

Cain P, Treiman D: The DOT as a source of occupational data. American Sociologist Review 46:253–278, 1981

Cohen LH, Towbes LC, Flocco R: Effects of induced mood on self-reported life events and perceived and received social support. J Pers Soc Psychol 55:669–674, 1988

Dohrenwend BP: Stressful life events and psychopathology: some issues of theory and method, in Stress and Mental Disorder. Edited by Barrett JF, Rose RM, Klerman GL. New York, Raven, 1979, pp 1–15

Dohrenwend BP, Shrout PE, Link BG, et al: Overview and initial results from a risk factor study of depression and schizophrenia, in Stress and Mental Disorder. Edited by Barrett JE, Rose RM. New York, Guilford, 1986, pp 1–15

Dohrenwend BP, Levav I, Shrout PE, et al: Socioeconomic status and psychiatric disorders: the causation selection issue. Science 255:946–952, 1992

Dohrenwend BP, Raphael KG, Schwartz S, et al: The structured event probe and narrative rating method (SEPRATE) for measuring stressful life events, in Handbook of Stress: Theoretical and Clinical Aspects, 2nd Edition. Edited by Goldberger L, Bresnitz S. New York, Free Press, 1993, pp 174–199

Dohrenwend BS, Dohrenwend BP (eds): Stressful Life Events: Their Nature and Effects. New York, Wiley, 1974

Dohrenwend BS, Dohrenwend BP: Life stress and illness: formulation of the issues, in Stressful Life Events and Their Contexts. Edited by Dohrenwend BS, Dohrenwend BP. New York, Neale Watson Academic, 1981, pp 1–27 (republished by Rutgers University Press, New Brunswick, NJ, 1983)

Dohrenwend BS, Krasnoff L, Askenasy AR, et al: The psychiatric epidemiology research interview life events scale, in Handbook of Stress: Theoretical and Clinical Aspects. Edited by Goldberger L, Breznitz S. New York, Free Press, 1982, pp 332–363

Fischer C: To Dwell Among Friends: Personal Networks in Town and City. Chicago, IL, University of Chicago Press, 1982

Hammen C, Davila J, Brown G, et al: Psychiatric history and stress: predictors of severity of unipolar depression. J Abnorm Psychol 101:45–52, 1992

Hirschfeld RMA, Klerman GL, Clayton PJ, et al: Assessing personality: effects of the depressive state on trait measurement. Am J Psychiatry 140:695–699, 1983

Jenkins CD, Rosenman RH, Friedman M: Development of an objective psychological test for the determination of the coronary-prone behavior pattern. J Chronic Dis 20:371–379, 1967

Jourard SM: Self-Disclosure: An Experimental Analysis of the Transparent Self. New York, Wiley-Interscience, 1971

Leff J, Vaughn C: The role of maintenance therapy and relatives' expressed emotion in relapse of schizophrenia: a 2-year follow-up. Br J Psychiatry 139:102–104, 1981

Levenson H: Multidimensional locus of control in psychiatric patients. J Consult Clin Psychol 47:397–404, 1972

Lewinsohn PM, Hoberman HM, Rosenbaum M: A prospective study of risk factors for unipolar depression. J Abnorm Psychol 97:251–264, 1988

Link BG, Dohrenwend BP, Skodol AE: Socioeconomic status and schizophrenia: noisome occupational characteristics as a risk factor. American Sociological Review 51:242–258, 1986

Link BG, Cullen FT, Struening E, et al: A modified labeling theory approach to mental disorders: an empirical assessment. American Sociological Review 54:400–423, 1989

Lukoff D, Snyder K, Ventura J, et al: Life events, familial stress, and coping in the developmental course of schizophrenia. Schizophr Bull 10:258–292, 1984

McGuffin P, Katz R, Bebbington P: Hazard, heredity and depression: a family study. J Psychiatr Res 21:365–375, 1987

Miller SM: When is a little information a dangerous thing: coping with stressful events by monitoring vs blunting, in Coping and Health: Proceedings of a NATO Conference. Edited by Levine S, Ursin H. New York, Plenum, 1980, pp 145–170

Norman RMG, Malla AK: Stressful life events and schizophrenia, I: a review of the research. Br J Psychiatry 162:161–166, 1993

Orvaschel HO, Thompson WD, Belanger A, et al: Comparison of the family history method to direct interview: factors affecting the diagnosis of depression. J Affect Disord 4:49–59, 1982

Paykel ES: Life stress and psychiatric disorder: applications of the clinical approach, in Stressful Life Events: Their Nature and Effects. Edited by Dohrenwend BS, Dohrenwend BP. New York, Wiley, 1974, pp 135–149

Pearlin LI, Johnson JS: Marital status, life strains and depression. American Sociological Review 42:704–715, 1977

Rabkin JG, Struening EL: Life events, stress and illness. Science 194:1013–1020, 1976

Raphael KG: Recall bias: a proposal for assessment and control. Int J Epidemiol 16:167–170, 1987

Raphael KG, Dohrenwend BP: Self-disclosure and mental health: a problem of confounded measurement. J Abnorm Psychol 96:214–217, 1987

Rotter JB: Generalized expectancies of internal versus external control of reinforcement. Psychological Monographs 80:609, 1966

Shrout PE, Link BG, Dohrenwend BP, et al: Characterizing life events as risk factors for depression: the role of fateful loss events. J Abnorm Psychol 98:460–467, 1989

Skodol AE, Williams JBW, Spitzer RL, et al: Identifying common errors in the use of DSM-III through diagnostic supervision. Hosp Community Psychiatry 35:251–255, 1984

Spence JT, Helmreich R: Masculinity and Femininity: Their Psychological Dimensions, Correlates and Antecedents. Austin, University of Texas Press, 1978

Steinberg H, Durell J: A stressful social situation as a precipitant of schizophrenic symptoms: an epidemiological study. Br J Psychiatry 114:1097–1105, 1968

U.S. Department of Labor: Dictionary of Occupational Titles. Washington, DC, U.S. Government Printing Office, 1977

Wyler AR, Masuda M, Holmes TH: The seriousness of illness rating scale. J Psychosom Res 11:363–374, 1968

Zubin J, Spring B: Vulnerability: a new view of schizophrenia. J Abnorm Psychol 86:103–126, 1977

Chapter 3

Stress, Dopamine, and Schizophrenia: Evidence for a Stress-Diathesis Model

Alan Breier, M.D.

Stress appears to play a role in the pathophysiology of most psychiatric illnesses. One of the most compelling pathophysiologic models for psychiatric illnesses is the so-called stress-diathesis model. This model posits that an abnormal biological substrate (diathesis) is acted on by stress to produce or exacerbate symptoms and signs of the illness. Following from this model, it is predicted that stress-reducing treatments (both behavioral and pharmacologic) would improve the course of illness. Direct evidence for an abnormal diathesis for major psychiatric illness, however, has not been produced.

Schizophrenia is arguably the most severe of all of the psychiatric disorders and, from a public health perspective, is one of the worst illnesses affecting humankind. It is a common disorder, with approximately 1% of the population affected. The illness typically begins early in life (i.e., the second or third decade) and for many patients runs a chronic lifelong course. The cost of schizophrenia for lost productivity and treatment is approximately $30 million per year in the United States (Andrews et al. 1985; McGuire 1991). Last, schizophrenia is a potentially lethal illness, as demonstrated by a 20% earlier mortality rate than the nonschizophrenic population, which includes, but is not totally explained by, a 10% suicide rate (Breier and Astrachan 1984).

This chapter examines clinical studies relevant to the role of stress in the course of illness and outcome of schizophrenia.

A revised version of the dopamine hypothesis that emphasizes a neural-circuits framework is presented. Preclinical data about the effects of stress on dopamine function are reviewed. A neuro-anatomical hypothesis is proposed that suggests that stress-related effects on dopamine regulation are involved in the pathophysiology of schizophrenia. In addition, methodological issues inherent in stress-induction research for major psychiatric illnesses are discussed. Last, the results of an experiment that tests the stress-related dopamine dysregulation hypothesis is presented.

STRESS EFFECTS IN SCHIZOPHRENIA: EVIDENCE FROM CLINICAL STUDIES

Evidence from four lines of clinical research supports the role of stress in the pathophysiology of schizophrenia: 1) the relationship between discrete stressful life events and relapse, 2) the relationship between chronic interpersonal stress and relapse, 3) the effects of stress-reducing behavioral approaches on course of illness, and 4) the effects of stress-reducing pharmacologic treatments on psychotic symptoms.

Stressful Life Events and Psychotic Relapse

Although there is a long history of research into the relationship between discrete stressful life events and the onset and exacerbation of schizophrenia, much of the earlier work is flawed by methodological shortcomings. There are six methodological issues that are important in examining the relationship between life events and relapses in schizophrenic patients: 1) prospective design, 2) appropriate control group (e.g., nonrelapsing schizophrenic patients), 3) classification of life events blindly as "independent" of the relapse (i.e., clarify that the life event was not caused by the relapse), 4) use of a comprehensive life event inventory that includes "minor" events as well as "major" events (see later in this section), 5) use of operationalized definitions of relapse with validated criteria for when the relapse began, and 6) accountability for neuroleptic compliance and other non-stress-related factors that could cause relapses (e.g., drug use).

There are very few studies that have accounted for all or most of these methodological factors. Of those that have, a significant relationship between stressful life events and relapse in schizophrenic patients has been found. In a controlled, prospective study, Ventura et al. (1989) found that there were significantly more independent life events in the month preceding psychotic relapse in schizophrenic outpatients. In a subsequent study, Ventura et al. (1992) showed that neuroleptic medication produces a prophylactic effect to stress-induced relapse and suggested that neuroleptics may raise a patient's threshold of vulnerability to relapse. Although a significant relationship between stressful life events and subsequent psychotic relapse was found, the overall strength of the relationship is relatively modest, suggesting that factors in addition to stress should be considered as possible triggers to relapse.

In a 1-year prospective study of schizophrenic outpatients, Malla et al. (1990) examined the relationship between psychotic relapse and both major and minor events. Minor events (or "daily hassles") include difficulties related to common circumstances such as "not enough money for clothing," "family responsibilities," and "transportation problems" (Kanner et al. 1981). The authors found that relapsed patients had experienced significantly more independent major and minor life events compared with nonrelapsing patients and that there were more events in the period immediately preceding relapse than at other times during the year-long study period. When major and minor events were considered separately, the relationship to relapse was less strong, which underlines the importance of considering minor as well as major life events.

Moreover, in another study, Malla and colleagues found that schizophrenic patients had greater levels of distress associated with minor events than with major events (Norman and Malla 1991). These data suggest that schizophrenic patients have unique and idiosyncratic responses to stress.

Chronic Interpersonal Stress

Exposure to chronic interpersonal stress, such as high expressed emotion, has been shown to predict relapse in schizophrenic patients. From 1962 to 1987, there have been 12 controlled studies of expressed emotion (see Mintz et al. 1987). In these studies, the number of relapses over a fixed interval (typically 9–12 months) for schizophrenic patients residing in households with high expressed emotion was compared with the number of patients residing in households with low expressed emotion. The results from the 12 studies indicated that there was a cumulative relapse rate of 53% among patients residing in households with high expressed emotion as compared with a 23% relapse rate in patients residing in households with low expressed emotion. Current research is investigating the determinants of this phenomenon. Schreiber et al. (in press) provided support for the hypothesis that expressed emotion may not be a parental trait but rather a product of the relationship between the ill offspring and the parent.

Stress-Reducing Treatments

Behavioral treatments that lower the levels of ambient stress in the environment decrease relapse rates and improve symptom and functioning outcomes (Falloon et al. 1985; Hogarty et al. 1986). Falloon et al. (1985) assessed a psychoeducationally based family management treatment module that emphasized problem-solving techniques that lowered levels of family stress and tension. This module was compared with traditional case management over a 9-month period. Patients assigned to family management had significantly fewer relapses and hospitalizations, lower levels of symptoms, and higher levels of functioning and required less neuroleptic medication than the comparison group. Hogarty et al. (1986) assessed the efficacy of social skills training and psychoeducational approaches in families with high expressed emotion and found that relapse rates were significantly improved with these treatments.

Treatment with pharmacologic agents, such as benzodiazepines, that have a direct action on neurochemical systems that mediate stress effects and anxiety improves the outcome of schizophrenia. A comprehensive review of this literature is provided elsewhere (Wolkowitz and Pickar 1991). In summary, a review of 30 double-blind trials found that benzodiazepines resulted in a significant improvement in one-third to one-half of schizophrenic patients treated.

Thus, these studies support the role of stress in the pathophysiology of schizophrenia. As noted earlier, however, the "diathesis" on which stress and stress-reducing treatments act has not been elucidated. In the following sections, altered dopaminergic function is examined as the putative diathesis in the stress-diathesis model of schizophrenia.

DOPAMINE HYPOTHESIS OF SCHIZOPHRENIA REVISITED: ROLE OF CORTICAL–SUBCORTICAL CIRCUITS

The original dopamine hypothesis of schizophrenia stated that hyperactive dopamine activity was responsible for the primary symptoms and signs of the illness. Simple, unidimensional models (i.e., too much or too little dopamine) have been replaced with more sophisticated models that emphasize dysregulation of dopamine function and implicate interactions between dopamine neurons and other neurotransmitter systems (e.g., γ-aminobutyric acid [GABA], glutamate) that act to modulate dopamine firing rates. These more complex models have led to an emphasis on neuroanatomical circuits (i.e., a series of different brain regions that are neurochemically and functionally linked). The perspective of considering neurochemical deficits in a neural-circuits framework has reoriented theoretical and experimental approaches to the pathophysiology of schizophrenia.

A dysfunction in cortical-subcortical circuits leading to altered subcortical dopamine function in schizophrenia has been proposed (Davis et al. 1991; Grace 1991; Pickar et al. 1990; Weinberger 1987). Evidence from clinical studies for such dysfunction includes a negative relationship found between cerebrospinal fluid levels of homovanillic acid (HVA), a major circulating metabolite of dopamine, and prefrontal cortical atrophy (Doran et al. 1987). In addition, a positive relationship has been reported between cerebrospinal fluid HVA concentrations and activation during frontal cognitive tasks in schizophrenic patients (Weinberger et al. 1988).

In a magnetic resonance imaging (MRI) study, we reported that schizophrenic patients, in comparison with control subjects, had significant reductions in total prefrontal cortical and limbic structure (i.e., amygdala and hippocampus) volumes (Breier et al. 1992a). When prefrontal cortex volumes were segmented into gray and white matter, it was learned that the schizophrenic patients had volume reductions in white matter (i.e., the tracks leading to and coming away from cortex) and that there was a positive relationship between white matter reductions and limbic structure volumes. These data support the hypothesis that the prefrontal cortex may be functionally "disconnected" from subcortical structures in schizophrenic patients and that there may be an abnormal prefrontal-limbic neural circuit in this illness.

DOPAMINE, STRESS, AND THE PREFRONTAL CORTEX

There are three major dopamine projections in the mammalian brain that have been of interest to scientists investigating schizophrenia: nigrostriatal projections, which innervate the basal ganglia (principally the caudate and putamen); mesolimbic projections, which innervate limbic structures (e.g., amygdala, accumbens); and mesocortical projections, which principally innervate the prefrontal cortex, cingulate, and entorhinal areas. Although all dopamine projections are sensitive to stress, the mesocortical projections to prefrontal cortex are preferentially activated during stress exposure, with greater degrees of dopamine turnover during stress exposure than all other dopamine projections (Thierry et al. 1976). There is evidence that this exaggerated response to stress may play an important modulatory role on subcortical dopamine activity.

Several, but not all, preclinical studies have shown that experimentally induced lesions of prefrontal cortex dopamine neurons produce increased subcortical dopamine activity (Carter 1982; Deutch et al. 1990; Haroutunian et al. 1988; Lecceses and Lyness 1987). Interestingly, this so-called Pycock effect (named after the investigator whose laboratory reported this phenomenon) appears to be more consistently produced when animals are examined during stressful perturbation. Deutch et al. (1990) found that prefrontal dopamine lesions failed to affect subcortical dopamine activity during the resting state. However, when animals where exposed to stress, significantly greater elevations in subcortical dopamine activity were found in the prefrontally lesioned animals than in the nonlesioned control animals. Jaskiw et al. (1990) reported similar findings with anatomical lesions of prefrontal cortex. These data suggest that cortically induced deficits in subcortical dopamine regulation are "uncovered" during stress because of the enhanced demands stress places on regulatory mechanisms.

STRESS–RELATED DYSREGULATION OF DOPAMINE FUNCTION: CORTICAL–SUBCORTICAL HYPOTHESIS OF SCHIZOPHRENIA

The hypothesis that emerges from the studies cited earlier is that stress-induced dysregulation of dopamine function is involved in the pathophysiology of schizophrenia and that this deficit occurs because of a failure of normal cortical modulation of subcortical dopaminergic activity. Thus, dysregulated subcortical dopaminergic function is the proposed diathesis in the stress-diathesis model of schizophrenia.

As noted in the preclinical studies mentioned earlier (Deutch et al. 1990; Jaskiw et al. 1990), deficits of neurotransmitter regulation are more likely to be "uncovered" when the systems in question are exposed to stress, as opposed to being studied in the resting state. Thus, we conducted an experiment to test the above hypothesis by assessing dopaminergic function in schizophrenic patients during stress exposure and then determining if putative stress-induced alterations were related to abnormalities in prefrontal cortex. The proposed hypothesis predicts that alterations in dopamine function would be either relatively mild or not observed in the nonstressed state, but they would be fully manifested during stress exposure. Before presenting these data, methodological issues of stress-induction research in schizophrenic patients are reviewed in the next section.

METHODOLOGICAL ISSUES OF STRESS–INDUCTION RESEARCH IN SCHIZOPHRENIA

There are several methodological issues involved in developing stress-induction paradigms for studies of major psychiatric illnesses. As shown in Table 3–1, there are three types of stress: cognitive, affective, and physical. It is suggested that the type of stress to be induced should be predicated on the specific research questions and diagnostic group. A central concept in this scheme is that qualitative (i.e., which type of stress induction is desired) as opposed to solely quantitative (i.e., how strong will the stress response be) judgments should be considered in designing a stress-induction paradigm.

Developing stress-induction paradigms for studies of schizophrenia poses unique challenges. Schizophrenia is commonly associated with cognitive deficits. Thus, use of a cognitive stressor may introduce mental performance confounds that may invalidate comparisons between cognitively impaired schizophrenic patients and cognitively intact control subjects. In addition, motivational deficits, asociality, and lack of social drive are common characteristics of many schizophrenic patients, particularly those with negative symptom syndromes. Thus, the use of an affective stressor may confound comparisons of schizophrenic patients with control subjects because affective stressors often rely on the subject's desire to please the experimenter or on an internal drive to succeed, both of which may be lacking in schizophrenic patients.

Physical stressors, on the other hand, have the advantages of not being associated with mental performance confounds and the degree of stress induced not being contingent on dynamics between experimenter and subject or on motivational characteristics of the subject. Thus, there is less variance in the level of stress that is induced in patients and control subjects. In addition, many physical stressors tend to produce a stronger neurochemical response with relatively less individual variability than cognitive and affective stressors. Also, physical stressors are well suited for designs requiring repeated exposure because they are accompanied by relatively low levels of habituation.

Table 3–1. Strategies for psychiatric stress-induction research				
Types of stress	Mechanism for stress induction	Advantages (+) and disadvantages (–)	Clinical application	Examples of stressors
Cognitive	Increase cognitive load/interference	+ Anatomical specificity – Performance bias – Habituation	Alzheimer's; cognitive deficits of other illness	Neuropsychological tests (e.g., Stroop, Raven's)
Affective	Induce negative emotional states (e.g., embarrassment, failure, anxiety)	+ Strong emotional response – Much individual variability – Rapid habituation – Ethical considerations	Depression, anxiety disorders, PTSD; deficits of other affective illness	Criticism, shock threat
Physical	Disrupt physiological homeostasis	+ Strong physiological response + No performance bias + Decreased individual variability + Decreased habituation – May lack anatomical specificity	Lacks illness specificity; probe neurochemical/anatomical hypotheses	Glucose deprivation

Note. PTSD = posttraumatic stress disorder.

NOVEL GLUCOSE–DEPRIVATION PARADIGM FOR SCHIZOPHRENIA STUDIES

A physical stressor that has several advantages for examining stress effects on dopamine function in schizophrenia is glucose deprivation. Glucose deprivation is a classical central nervous system stressor and is extensively characterized in both preclinical and clinical stress studies. Because glucose is the primary energy source of the central nervous system, its deprivation causes potent perturbation throughout the brain. In addition, glucose deprivation has strong effects on dopamine function, including increasing dopamine turnover (Agardh et al. 1979; Heyes et al. 1990; Sauter et al. 1983) and increasing brain (Sauter et al. 1983) and plasma (Breier 1989) levels of the dopamine metabolite HVA. Glucose deprivation also has the advantages mentioned above in that it is not associated with mental performance confounds and is not contingent on the motivational or cognitive status of the subject.

The most commonly used glucose deprivation paradigm is insulin-induced hypoglycemia. Insulin acts to decrease plasma glucose levels so that less glucose is available to the brain. We have developed an alternative paradigm that involves infusion of pharmacologic doses of 2-deoxyglucose (2DG) (Breier et al. 1988, 1991a). 2DG is a glucose analog that is transported into the brain cells and then phosphorylated in the same manner as glucose itself. The phosphorylated form of 2DG (i.e., 2DG6P), however, cannot be metabolized and accumulates, which prevents the normal metabolism of glucose (Horton et al. 1973). Thus, 2DG competitively inhibits the intracellular usage of glucose, which creates a state of "intracellular hypoglycemia." When given in doses sufficient to block glucose metabolism, 2DG produces a clinical state that is similar to insulin-induced hypoglycemia (Bachelard 1971; Horton et al. 1973; Sols and Crane 1954).

We have conducted several preclinical and clinical studies of the effects of pharmacologic doses of 2DG. 2DG causes a robust increase in local cerebral blood flow in several brain regions, including those areas that have been implicated in cortical-subcortical neuroanatomical hypotheses of schizophrenia (e.g., prefrontal cortex, anterior cingulate, basal ganglia, and thala-

mus) (Breier et al. 1993a). The 2DG stressor has very strong stim-
ulatory effects on two classical stress systems: the pituitary-
adrenal and adrenomedullary systems (Breier et al. 1991a,
1992b). In addition, 2DG produces neuroendocrine effects that
differentiate schizophrenic patients from healthy control subjects
(Breier and Buchanan 1992).

STRESS–INDUCED DYSREGULATION
OF DOPAMINE: RELATIONSHIP TO
PREFRONTAL CORTEX

To test directly the hypothesis that schizophrenic patients have
stress-related dysregulation of dopamine function that is associated with deficits in prefrontal-subcortical connections, we have
used the 2DG paradigm to assess the effects of stress on levels of
the dopamine metabolite HVA in schizophrenic patients and
healthy control subjects. We also have used MRI-derived morphological characteristics of the prefrontal cortex to determine if
possible stress-related alterations in plasma HVA are related to
the prefrontal cortex abnormalities. These findings, summarized
here, have been presented in more detail elsewhere (Breier et al.
1993b).

Methods

Eighteen schizophrenic patients (ages 32 ± 5 years; 3 females) and
11 healthy control subjects (ages 26 ± 5 years; 4 females) participated in the 2DG protocol; 15 of the 18 patients underwent MRIs.
Patients were all chronic outpatients (12 ± 6 years of illness).
DSM-III-R (American Psychiatric Association 1987) diagnoses
were made in the context of a best-estimate diagnostic meeting,
using all available sources of information including a structured
diagnostic interview (Spitzer et al. 1990). Control subjects were
recruited from the general population and did not have current
or past psychiatric illnesses as determined from the diagnostic
interview. Both patients and control subjects were in good physical health.

2DG protocol. Each subject had 2 test days: an active 2DG day and a placebo-infusion day. The study was conducted double-blind, and the order of test days was randomized. 2DG doses were 50 mg/kg mixed in 100 ml of isotonic saline. Placebo consisted of comparable volumes of isotonic saline alone. Subjects fasted from midnight prior to each test day and reported to the clinic between 8:00 A.M. and 9:00 A.M. for the study. An intravenous catheter was inserted into the antecubital fossa of each subject and kept patent with a slow drip of normal saline. After an hour acclimation period and collection of baseline blood samples for HVA and cortisol levels, behavioral ratings, and physiological parameters, either placebo or 2DG was infused over the subsequent 30 minutes. Data (bloods, behavioral ratings, and physiological parameters) were then collected over the subsequent 2 hours. At that time, the intravenous catheter was removed, and the study ended.

MRI protocol. All scans were performed with a 2-T Siemens Magnetom Scanner operating at 1.5 T. After obtaining a sagittal scout film to adjust head tilt and establish scanning coordinates, the whole brain was evaluated in the coronal plane with 3-mm contiguous (no gap) slices using high-resolution spin-echo technique with a TR of 600 μsec and a TE of 17 μsec, with two excitations and a matrix size of 265 by 256 pixels. Morphological analyses were performed using a Loats Image Analysis System (Loats, Inc., Westminster, Maryland; Loats et al. 1988). A rules-based system to identify the boundaries of the frontal cortex was used (Breier et al. 1992a). Total volume was calculated from area measurements obtained from each slice.

Results

2DG effects on plasma HVA. Both schizophrenic patients and control subjects had significant increases in plasma HVA levels compared with levels on the placebo-infusion test day (Table 3–2). The 2DG-related HVA increases in schizophrenic patients were significantly greater than those in control subjects (Figure 3–1). There was a trend for schizophrenic patients to have

Table 3–2.   Effects (mean ± SD) of 2-deoxyglucose (2DG)–induced metabolic perturbation on plasma homovanillic acid (ng/ml) in 11 healthy control subjects and 18 schizophrenic patients

Subjects	Baseline	+60 min	+90 min	+120 min	+150 min
Control subjects					
Placebo	10.7 ± 6.6	8.8 ± 5.5	7.9 ± 5.2	8.5 ± 5.0	7.5 ± 4.1
Active 2DG	8.9 ± 2.7	7.9 ± 2.3	8.2 ± 2.4	9.5 ± 2.8	9.3 ± 3.1
Schizophrenic patients					
Placebo	6.8 ± 2.9	5.9 ± 2.0	5.3 ± 1.9	5.2 ± 2.0	5.2 ± 2.1
Active 2DG	6.6 ± 1.4	6.7 ± 1.9	7.3 ± 1.8	8.1 ± 1.9	8.6 ± 2.3

Note.   Schizophrenia-active 2DG versus control-active 2DG: group: $F = 2.6$, df = 1,26, $P = .06$; group X time: $F = 3.5$, df = 4,23, $P = .01$. Drug (2DG and placebo) versus time: control subjects: $F = 8.9$, df = 4,4, $P = .30$; schizophrenic patients: $F = 8.9$, df = 4,14, $P = .001$.

lower plasma HVA levels on the placebo test day than did control subjects. 2DG caused robust increases in plasma cortisol levels in both patients and control subjects. There were, however, no significant differences in plasma cortisol levels between the groups (Figure 3–1). A subgroup of schizophrenic patients who were tested while receiving neuroleptic treatment were compared with drug-free schizophrenic patients, and it was found that neuroleptic treatment did not alter 2DG effects on plasma HVA and cortisol levels.

2DG-induced increases in plasma HVA were related to 2DG-induced increases in behavioral ratings of fatigue ($r = .47, P = .03$) and stress ($r = .42, P = .08$) and to plasma cortisol level increases ($r = .50, P = .03$).

2DG-induced HVA responses and frontal cortex. The prefrontal cortex total volumes (mean ± SD cc) of the patients in this study (left prefrontal cortex, $77.6 ± 14$; right prefrontal cortex, $81.3 ± 11$) were similar to those for the schizophrenic group who, as we previously reported, had significantly smaller total volumes than did matched healthy control subjects (Breier et al.

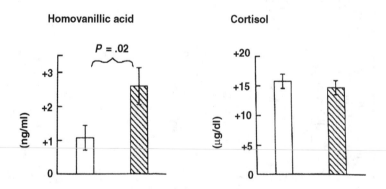

Figure 3–1. Comparison of 2-deoxyglucose stress-induced peak changes (mean ± SE) in plasma indices in 11 healthy control subjects *(open bar)* and 18 schizophrenic subjects *(striped bar)*. Peak changes = peak value minus baseline value.

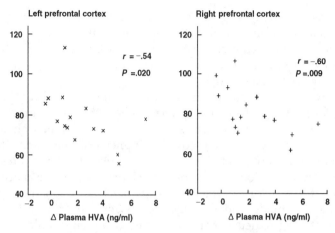

Figure 3–2. Relationship between prefrontal cortex volume and 2-deoxyglucose-induced change in plasma homovanillic acid (HVA) in schizophrenia.

1992a). There was a significant inverse relationship between 2DG-induced elevations in plasma HVA levels and right and left prefrontal cortex total volumes (Figure 3–2). Thus, those patients with the smallest prefrontal cortices had the largest 2DG-related increases in plasma HVA.

Discussion

The two major findings of this study are that schizophrenic patients, in comparison with control subjects, have significantly greater 2DG-induced elevations in plasma HVA concentrations and that these elevations are significantly and inversely related to prefrontal cortex size.

Interestingly, plasma HVA levels in schizophrenic patients were not significantly elevated on the placebo test days (they were actually somewhat lower than control levels). Thus, as in the work of Deutch et al. (1990) and others (Jaskiw et al. 1990) cited earlier, stress exposure was required to "uncover" what appears to be a deficit in dopamine regulation. The fact that

2DG-related changes in plasma cortisol levels were not different between the groups suggests that schizophrenia is not related to global or nonspecific abnormalities in the stress response but rather may have a relatively specific deficit related to stress effects on dopamine function.

Chronic neuroleptic treatment did not attenuate 2DG effects on plasma HVA. Thus, these data suggest that stress-induced dysregulation of dopamine is not "corrected" by neuroleptic treatment and provides a theoretical framework to explain why patients who are treated with neuroleptics still have stress-related exacerbations of symptoms. Hypotheses of the mechanism of action of neuroleptic drugs, such as depolarization blockade (Chiodo and Bunney 1983; White and Wang 1983), would have predicted that neuroleptic treatment would block stress-related increases in dopamine function. If the plasma HVA data from this report reflect dopamine function in brain (for a discussion of this issue, see Breier et al. 1993b), a modification in theories of neuroleptic drug action may be indicated.

The inverse relationship between 2DG stress-induced elevations in plasma HVA levels and prefrontal cortex volumes is supportive of the hypothesis that a failure of normal prefrontal cortical inhibition of subcortical dopamine function may be responsible for the elevated stress-induced increases in plasma HVA levels in the schizophrenic patients. We are currently working on new paradigms that combine stressors, such as 2DG, with direct measures of central dopamine function (e.g., displacement of ^{11}C-labeled raclopride binding and perturbations of ^{18}F-labeled dopa) using positron-emission tomography.

In conclusion, several lines of evidence were examined that suggest a pathophysiologic hypothesis of schizophrenia that involves stress-induced dysregulation of subcortical dopamine activity that may occur because of a disruption in normal cortical-subcortical connections.

REFERENCES

Agardh C-D, Carlsson A, Lindqvist M, et al: The effect of pronounced hypoglycemia on monoamine metabolism in rat brain. Diabetes 28:804–809, 1979

American Psychiatric Association: Diagnostic and Statistical Manual of Mental Disorders, 3rd Edition, Revised. Washington, DC, American Psychiatric Association, 1987

Andrews G, Hall W, Goldstein G, et al: The economic costs of schizophrenia: implications for public policy. Arch Gen Psychiatry 42: 537–543, 1985

Bachelard HS: Deoxyglucose and brain glycolysis. J Neurochem 18:213–222, 1971

Breier A: Experimental approaches to human stress research: assessment of neurobiological mechanisms of stress in volunteers and psychiatric patients. Biol Psychiatry 26:438–462, 1989

Breier A, Astrachan BM: Characterization of schizophrenic patients who commit suicide. Am J Psychiatry 141:206–209, 1984

Breier A, Buchanan RW: The effects of metabolic stress on plasma progesterone in healthy volunteers and schizophrenic patients. Life Sci 51:1527–1534, 1992

Breier A, Wolkowitz OM, Rappaport M, et al: Metabolic stress effects in normal volunteers and schizophrenic patients. Psychopharmacol Bull 24:431–433, 1988

Breier A, Davis OR, Buchanan RW: Alprazolam attenuates metabolic stress-induced neuroendocrine and behavioral effects in humans. Psychopharmacology (Berl) 104:479–484, 1991a

Breier A, Wolkowitz OM, Pickar D: Stress and schizophrenia, in Advances in Neuropsychiatry and Psychopharmacology, Vol 1: Schizophrenia Research. Edited by Tamminga CA, Schulz SC. New York, Raven, 1991b, pp 141–152

Breier A, Buchanan RW, Elkashef A, et al: Brain morphology and schizophrenia: an MRI study of limbic, prefrontal cortex and caudate structures. Arch Gen Psychiatry 49:921–926, 1992a

Breier A, Davis O, Buchanan RW, et al: Effects of alprazolam on pituitary-adrenal and catecholaminergic responses to metabolic stress in humans. Biol Psychiatry 32:880–890, 1992b

Breier A, Crane AM, Kennedy C, et al: The effects of pharmacologic doses of 2-deoxy-D-glucose on local cerebral blood flow in the awake, unrestrained rat. Brain Res 618:277–282, 1993a

Breier A, Davis OR, Buchanan RW, et al: Effects of metabolic perturbation on plasma homovanillic acid in schizophrenia: relationship to prefrontal cortex volume. Arch Gen Psychiatry 50:541–550, 1993b

Carter CJ: Topographical distribution of possible glutamatergic pathways from the frontal cortex to the striatum and substantia nigra in rats. Neuropharmacology 21:383–393, 1982

Chiodo LA, Bunney BS: Typical and atypical neuroleptics: differential effects of chronic administration on the activity of A9 and A10 midbrain dopaminergic neurons. J Neurosci 3:1607–1619, 1983

Davis KL, Kahn RS, Ko G, et al: Dopamine in schizophrenia: a review and reconceptualization. Am J Psychiatry 148:1474–1486, 1991

Deutch AY, Clark WA, Roth RH: Prefrontal cortical dopamine depletion enhances the responsiveness of mesolimbic dopamine neurons to stress. Brain Res 521:311–315, 1990

Doran AR, Boronow J, Weinberger DR, et al: Structural brain pathology in schizophrenia revisited: prefrontal cortex pathology is inversely correlated with cerebrospinal fluid levels of homovanillic acid. Neuropsychopharmacology 1:25–32, 1987

Falloon IRH, Boyd JL, McGill CW, et al: Family management in the prevention of morbidity of schizophrenia: clinical outcome of a two-year longitudinal study. Arch Gen Psychiatry 43:887–896, 1985

Grace AA: Phasic versus tonic dopamine release and the modulation of dopamine system responsivity: a hypothesis for the etiology of schizophrenia. Neuroscience 41:1–24, 1991

Haroutunian V, Knott P, Davis KL: Effects of mesocortical dopaminergic lesions upon subcortical dopaminergic function. Psychopharmacol Bull 24:341–344, 1988

Heyes MP, Papagapiou M, Leonard C, et al: Brain and plasma quinolinic acid in profound insulin-induced hypoglycemia. J Neurochem 54:1027–1033, 1990

Hogarty GE, Anderson CM, Reiss DJ, et al: Family psychoeducation, social skills training and maintenance chemotherapy in the aftercare treatment of schizophrenia. Arch Gen Psychiatry 43:633–641, 1986

Horton RW, Meldrum BS, Bachelard HS: Enzymic and cerebral metabolic effects of 2-deoxy-D-glucose. J Neurochem 21:507–520, 1973

Jaskiw GE, Karoum FK, Weinberger DR: Persistent elevations in dopamine and its metabolites in the nucleus accumbens after mild subchronic stress in rats with ibotenic acid lesions of the medial prefrontal cortex. Brain Res 534:263–272, 1990

Kanner AD, Coyne JC, Schaefer C, et al: Comparisons of two modes of stress measurement: daily hassles and uplifts versus major life events. J Behav Med 4:1–39, 1981

Lecceses AP, Lyness WH: Lesions of dopamine neurons in the medial prefrontal cortex: effects on self-administration of amphetamine and dopamine synthesis in the brain of the rat. Neuropharmacology 26:1303–1308, 1987

Loats HL, Lloyd DG, Pittenger M, et al: Biomedical image analysis applications, in Imaging Techniques in Biology and Medicine. Edited by Conklin JJ, Swenberg CE. New York, Academic Press, 1988, pp 1–75

Malla AK, Cortese L, Shaw TS, et al: Life events and relapse in schizophrenia: a one year prospective study. Soc Psychiatry Psychiatr Epidemiol 25:221–224, 1990

McGuire TG: Measuring the economic costs of schizophrenia. Schizophr Bull 17:375–388, 1991

Mintz LI, Liberman RP, Miklowitz DJ, et al: Expressed emotion: a call for partnership among relatives, patients, and professionals. Schizophr Bull 13:227–235, 1987

Norman RMG, Malla AK: Subjective stress in schizophrenic patients. Soc Psychiatry Psychiatr Epidemiol 26:212–216, 1991

Pickar D, Breier A, Hsiao JK, et al: Cerebrospinal fluid and plasma monoamine metabolites and their relation to psychosis. Arch Gen Psychiatry 47:641–648, 1990

Sauter A, Goldstein M, Engel J, et al: Effect of insulin on central catecholamine. Brain Res 260:330–333, 1983

Schreiber JL, Breier A, Pickar D: Expressed emotion: trait or state. Br J Psychiatry (in press)

Sols A, Crane RK: Substrate specificity of brain hexokinase. J Biol Chem 210:581–595, 1954

Spitzer RL, Williams JBW, Gibbon B, et al: Structured Clinical Interview for DSM-III-R. Washington, DC, American Psychiatric Press, 1990

Thierry AM, Tassin JP, Blanc G, et al: Selective activation of the mesocortical DA system by stress. Nature 263:242–244, 1976

Ventura J, Nuechterlein KH, Lukoff D, et al: A prospective study of stressful life events and schizophrenic relapse. J Abnorm Psychol 98:407–411, 1989

Ventura J, Nuechterlein KH, Hardesty JP, et al: Life events and schizophrenic relapse after withdrawal of medication. Br J Psychiatry 161:615–620, 1992

Weinberger DR: Implications of normal brain development for the pathogenesis of schizophrenia. Arch Gen Psychiatry 44:660–669, 1987

Weinberger DR, Berman KF, Illowsky BP: Physiological dysfunction of dorsolateral prefrontal cortex in schizophrenia, III: a new cohort and evidence for a monoaminergic mechanism. Arch Gen Psychiatry 45:609–615, 1988

White FJ, Wang RY: Differential effects of classical and atypical antipsychotic drugs on A9 and A10 dopamine neurons. Science 221:1054–1056, 1983

Wolkowitz OM, Pickar D: Benzodiazepines in the treatment of schizophrenia: a review and reappraisal. Am J Psychiatry 148:714–726, 1991

Chapter 4

Stress and the Course of Unipolar and Bipolar Disorders

Constance L. Hammen, Ph.D.

D oes stress cause psychiatric disorder? Much of the research that has addressed this provocative question over the past two decades has been concerned with depressive disorders or symptoms, the topic of the present chapter. Ultimately, the original question has proven to be too simple. The legacy of contemporary research on life stress and depression has been to make the question far more complicated and to necessitate more sophisticated methodologies. In addition, during this period, we have learned a great deal more about affective disorders, including bipolar disorders, posing additional challenges to our understanding of the role of stress. Therefore, I have two goals in this chapter. One is to refine some of the relevant questions in the stress disorder relationship, presenting recent research that addresses them. The second is to include bipolar disorders in the question of stress disorder associations and to discuss research exploring the role of stress in what has long been presumed to be a disorder of endogenous biological processes.

Before tackling these goals, however, some of the recent conceptual developments in stress-depression research and their implications are noted, and information about affective disorders emerging from recent studies is presented. These discussions are not intended to be comprehensive reviews of the topics, but serve as background for identifying new directions in the kinds of questions that are relevant to the stress disorder process.

RECENT CONCEPTUALIZATIONS OF THE STRESS–DEPRESSION RELATIONSHIP

Considerable research has established a significant association between depressive symptoms or diagnoses and stressful life events (Gotlib and Hammen 1992; Lloyd 1980; Thoits 1983). This association generally holds true for both clinical and community samples and for persons of all age groups. Much of the earlier research was flawed by limited assessment procedures, retrospective reporting, and failure to control current mood or reporting bias. Nevertheless, the essential finding that depressive symptoms or episodes are commonly preceded by the occurrence of negative life events has been established under conditions of rigorous control (e.g., Dohrenwend et al., Chapter 2, this volume; Shrout et al. 1989).

Despite such consistency of results, it is also true that only a small portion of the variance in depression is accounted for by stressors, and only some individuals have significant depressive reactions even to major stressors. Accordingly, recent efforts have turned to conceptual and methodological refinements to understand individual variation in stress reactivity. In particular, three themes have been emphasized by stress researchers in the past 15 years: appraisal processes, context, and coping and resources.

Appraisal Processes

It is now widely accepted that the impact of negative events is due not simply to their occurrence but rather to the ways in which they are construed. Richard Lazarus, in work that has evolved over several decades, has argued that stressors may be appraised as threats, or challenges, or as benign, depending on what the person thinks that the stakes are (primary appraisal); appraisal of the coping options (secondary appraisal) figures importantly in one's emotional reactions to stressors (e.g., Lazarus and Folkman 1984, 1987). The person's reactions to stressful life events or even "daily hassles" is, therefore, a dynamic process depending on the transaction between the person's appraisals and the actual environmental experiences.

Lazarus's formulations do not apply specifically to depression, but they are similar to those of Aaron Beck and attribution theorists, who emphasize the role of dysfunctional cognitions in depressive reactions (Abramson et al. 1978; Beck 1976). Beck has argued, for example, that negative interpretations of events that focus on pessimistic or self-critical appraisals will lead to depression. Similarly, Abramson et al. has emphasized that explanations of the causes of negative events that include internal, global, and stable attributions would lead to depressive reactions; that is, if a person interprets the cause of a negative life event to be something about the self that is unchanging and general, depression is likely to result.

Considerable research and analyses of these models have explored their strengths and limitations (e.g., Gotlib and Hammen 1992); despite their weaknesses, these diathesis-stress models of depression retain their importance. The diathesis specifically refers to tendencies toward negative cognitions about stressors. These models also concur in their emphasis that individual differences in appraisal help to account for why some individuals experience depression and others do not following objectively negative events. Additionally—and this is an important corollary—they emphasize that even objectively neutral or minor events may be misconstrued and viewed more negatively than their circumstances warrant. Thus, personal vulnerabilities based on previous learning experiences may lead to idiosyncratic appraisals that cause depressive reactions. This hypothesis makes it difficult simply to compare individuals on some metric of stress severity and to draw conclusions, because objective severity may not capture individually meaningful precipitants.

Context

The work of George Brown and his colleagues in London has been especially influential in pointing out the importance of studying the meaning of negative life events as reflected in the context of their occurrence. For both methodological and conceptual reasons, Brown and Harris (1978) developed interview methods of evaluating not just the occurrence of negative events, but also the circumstances surrounding the event. Consider the idea that a woman's pet dog died. If she checks the item on a question-naire of recent life events, its significance may be assumed to be the same for everyone who experiences the event. However, Brown's contextual threat method of assessment might determine that the woman is a widow whose only companion was the dog and that she has few social contacts or supports. When the entire context of the information is known, independent raters can then evaluate the "objective threat" or impact of the event in context and do so without knowledge of how the person actually reacted so as not to bias or inflate the association between events and emotional reactions.

Brown's work has also refined further elements of the "meaning" of events in terms of assessing the chronic strains (ongoing difficulties) the person lives with and the importance (commitment) the person might attach to particular roles. Episodic events that "match" the ongoing difficulties (e.g., son jailed against background of ongoing mother-son discord) or events that "match" prior commitment (e.g., someone who highly values the role of wife discovers her husband had an affair) are highly likely to lead to depression (Brown et al. 1987). Brown has further pursued the concept of meaning of events by observing that certain individuals may have particular early childhood adversities that create enduring vulnerabilities to experiencing depression when major negative events occur (e.g., Harris et al. 1986, 1987). The details of these complex formulations are not pursued here. Instead, the important implication of this body of work is the emphasis on the historical and current context for understanding individual differences in depressive reactions to negative life events.

It might be noted that other contemporary investigators have also explored contextual elements of depressive reactions. Their approach might be construed as a multivariate approach to the stress-depression relationship. Investigators such as Rudolph Moos and his colleagues and Peter Lewinsohn and his group assessed multiple variables such as cognitive constructs of self-concept and other appraisal styles, sociodemographic factors, marital strain, employment, and a host of resource and stress factors. The variables are entered into complex equations to predict depressive outcomes in large samples (e.g., Billings et al.

1983; Holahan and Moos 1991; Lewinsohn et al. 1988). Variations in the multiple elements of a person's life help to increase the predictability of depressive reactions.

Coping and Resources

In addition to attempting to assess the role of individual vulnerability and risk factors, contemporary investigators have argued that differences in resources available for coping with stressors play an important role in determining depressive reactions. Thus, social supports such as confidants and family as well as individual coping styles (problem-solving versus emotion-focused) have all been shown to moderate the effects of stressors on depression (e.g., Brown and Harris 1978; Swindle et al. 1989).

Summary

When we ask whether stress causes depression, we now know that it depends considerably on how a person construes an event and on the circumstances and consequences of the life event. What might be meaningful to one person and viewed as an important loss or depletion might be experienced as benign by another.

We might also note that although considerable research has attempted to understand the psychosocial vulnerabilities of an individual, we know relatively little about biological substrates of depression vulnerability in response to stress. A discussion of the possibilities is beyond the scope of this chapter, but I emphasize the need for studies of both constitutional-genetic and acquired biological vulnerabilities (e.g., Gold et al. 1988).

FEATURES OF AFFECTIVE DISORDERS AND IMPLICATIONS FOR STRESS THEORIES

A further complication to the stress-depression issue concerns elements of the disorders themselves. Increasing clarification of characteristics and correlates of affective disorders presents additional challenges to models of stress-depression that are overly simplistic. A full discussion of these issues is available elsewhere (for a review, see Gotlib and Hammen 1992). I note several such issues and their implications.

First, for the majority of individuals, affective disorders are recurrent if not chronic conditions. Although it has always been recognized that bipolar disorders are recurrent, the extent of relapse or chronic symptomatology even in treated populations is only recently recognized (e.g., Harrow et al. 1990). Moreover, we now recognize that the great majority of persons with major depressive episodes will have recurrences, and a substantial proportion display chronically elevated symptoms.

Second, mood disorders affect lives. Particularly for those with recurrent or chronic symptoms, the extent of impairment of functioning in major roles is enormous. Research on depression documents not only its impact on families and interpersonal relationships (Gotlib and Hammen 1992; Hammen 1991a) but also its toll in terms of work and personal morale. Indeed, even nonclinical levels of depression may contribute to debilities of functioning that are as severe as—or even more severe than—many chronic medical illnesses (Wells et al. 1989).

The implication of these two points is that mood disorders may create negative contexts; thus, stressful life events may happen to people in circumstances that are already adverse and diminished in supports and resources. Moreover, changing patterns of mood states and functioning create a dynamic, transactional process that may be poorly captured by cross-sectional designs or linear models.

Third, most studies of affective disorders, notably stress disorder studies, are really about relapse. Relatively few individuals have initial episodes, compared with those having recurrences. Most research on stress has not separated those having first episodes from those having later episodes, but it is possible, if not likely, that somewhat different factors predict the two. The role of stressors may therefore be somewhat different, depending on where an individual is in the course of the disorder. (This is discussed more extensively later.)

Fourth, affective disorders, especially unipolar depressions, are heterogeneous. It is likely that subtypes differ in etiological and course factors, and the role of stressors may vary accordingly. Additionally, the extent of comorbidity in affective disorders is enormous but rarely fully considered. Little research, for example, has pursued the question of whether stressors have different attributes or effects on groups that differ in coexisting conditions.

Finally, sociodemographic patterns in affective disorders present challenges to explanatory models, including those that emphasize the role of stressors. Young people and women, for instance, have excesses of affective disorders, especially depression (Klerman and Weissman 1989). Do stressful life events contribute differentially to groups differing in risk? If so, what are the mechanisms of such processes?

THE UCLA LONGITUDINAL STUDY OF STRESS AND AFFECTIVE DISORDERS

In view of the numerous challenges to the simplicity of the stress-depression question, I attempt in the remainder of the discussion to address more specific questions to illuminate some of the complexities of the link between stress and affective disorders. In addition, I attempt to address the question in bipolar samples, as well as unipolar, to learn more about the generalizability of the phenomenon to a disorder that has long been presumed to have an endogenous, biologically driven basis.

Methods of Study

Approximately 40 unipolar and 60 bipolar outpatients in the UCLA Neuropsychiatric Institute Affective Disorders Clinic (Michael Gitlin, M.D., director) were studied longitudinally to examine the role of psychosocial factors in the course of their affective disorders. These were consecutive admissions who agreed to be interviewed at 3-month intervals for up to 2 years. All were adults over age 18 and were diagnosed as having a primary affective disorder by using DSM-III-R (American Psychiatric Association 1987) criteria. They entered the study after attaining remission of symptoms or best clinical state if they tended to have elevated baseline symptoms.

Demographic details of samples vary according to different analyses and are described as required.

Patients continued regular psychiatrist visits and were evaluated for symptom status at each visit by their physician using systematic clinical records that ensured comparable information for all patients. However, they were interviewed separately by research staff every 3 months for information on life stress.

The interviews assessed life event occurrence in the period since the previous interview using a method based on George Brown's (Brown and Harris 1978) contextual threat measurement of stress as a way to minimize patients' potential reporting biases and forgetfulness. The interview uses standardized probes to obtain detailed information about the timing, nature, circumstances, expectedness of events, and resources available. A written narrative was prepared for each event by the interviewer, specifically omitting descriptions of the individual's reactions to the event. The narratives were then evaluated by a research team that made a rating of the "objective" threat, or severity, of the event in the context in which it occurred using a 5-point scale ranging from no threat to severe threat. The team members were blind to the person's symptom status. The team also rated the extent to which the event occurred independently of the person; the 5-point scale ranged from totally independent to totally dependent. From this scale, events could be simply classified as independent of or at least partly dependent on the person. Events specifically related to the person's affective illness or treatment (e.g., being hospitalized for an episode) were not included. Reliabilities of ratings for both objective threat and independence were highly significant (Ellicott et al. 1990; Hammen et al. 1989).

At the initial life stress interview, and at later follow-ups, certain personality questionnaires and measures were administered and are discussed as relevant.

IS TIMING OF BIPOLAR EPISODES RELATED TO STRESSORS?

 As has been noted previously, there is now a wealth of information indicating that stressors predict symptoms and precede episodes in many cases of unipolar depression. The status of stress in the bipolar disorders has been less extensively studied, and those studies that do exist are quite limited in their methodologies. For instance, several studies have interviewed patients about their stressors prior to their first depressive episode. Such studies generally indicated high levels of stressors preceding the initial onset—especially compared with later episodes—but patients may have been asked to recall over a substantial period of years (e.g., Bidzinska 1984; Dunner et al. 1979; Glassner et al. 1979; Patrick et al. 1978). Other studies indicated relatively high levels of stressors prior to the most recent (index) episode (e.g., Ambelas 1979; Kennedy et al. 1983) or among those with late versus early onset of disorder (Glassner and Haldipur 1983). In addition to the limitations imposed by retrospective assessment of stressors, the studies also differed in their definitions and measurement of stressors, making comparability difficult.

Prospective Study of Stress and Bipolar Episodes

Ellicott et al. (1990) studied 61 bipolar patients (28 men). Of these patients, 46 were bipolar I and the rest bipolar II (atypical bipolar); 32 experienced hypomania, mania, or major depression at some point during the year, and the rest were symptom free or had only mild symptoms. Events occurring in the 3 months prior to onset of episodes (or the middle 3 months for nonrelapsing patients) were identified. Survival analysis evaluated the relative hazard rates for relapse as a function of level of stress (Figure 4–1). Those experiencing the highest levels of stress had a relative hazard of 4.53 compared with lower levels of stress ($P < .001$). Patients who with and without histories of relapse were compared on intensity of medication regimen and medication compliance; there were no differences.

Thus, it appears that stressors are associated with increased risk for recurrence or relapse, even in aggressively medicated patients. This pattern certainly fits with what our patients tell us about their efforts to keep their lives as stress free as possible as a way of curtailing symptoms. However, we need to continue to study whether some patients with certain characteristics, or illness features, are more susceptible to stress than are others.

Susceptibility to Stressors in Bipolar Patients

Among those who relapsed were some whose symptoms occurred even following low levels of stressors, although some of
those exposed to high levels did not relapse. Swendsen et al.
(J. Swendsen et al., unpublished observations, June 1993) attempted to explore individual correlates of stress reactivity.
There are two hypotheses to consider. One is that bipolar patients
are more reactive to stressors earlier in the course of the disorder
than later. Indeed, Post (1992) argued this point and provided a
biochemical model of the development of endogenous processes
that may trigger episodes in the absence of stressors. A second
hypothesis, based on research from unipolar patients, suggests
that there are personality factors and personal characteristics that
make some people more vulnerable or sensitized to stressors,
whereas others may be more resilient.

Although our longitudinal project was not specifically developed to test these hypotheses, several variables were available to
explore these two approaches. For example, information about
number of prior episodes, age at onset, and family history of
psychopathology was abstracted from clinical interviews. Sev-

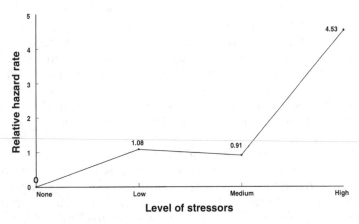

Figure 4–1. Relative hazard rate for bipolar relapse as a function of
stressor level. Adapted from Ellicott et al. 1990.

eral personality measures were completed by patients, including those used in the National Institute of Mental Health Collaborative Program on the Psychobiology of Depression (Hirschfeld et al. 1983): the Eysenck Personality Inventory (neuroticism and extraversion-introversion; Eysenck and Eysenck 1978); a measure of interpersonal dependency (the subscale of emotional reliance on other people from the Interpersonal Dependency Inventory; Hirschfeld et al. 1977); and the obsessionality subscale of the Lazare-Klerman-Armor scale (see Hirschfeld et al. 1989). These measures have variously predicted long-term negative outcomes in depressed patients and risk for onset (e.g., Andrews et al. 1990; Duggan et al. 1990; Hirschfeld et al. 1983, 1989). Additionally, the Personality Disorders Questionnaire (Hyler et al. 1988) was administered.

Bipolar patients were divided into those who relapsed during a 1-year follow-up period and those who did not relapse. These groups were subdivided into those who experienced high or low levels of stress based on 1-year objective threat totals, divided at the median. In the low stress group, comparisons between those who relapsed (who may be considered "vulnerable" or "reactive") and those who did not relapse indicated that none of the psychiatric history variables differed, whereas three of the five personality measures were significantly different. Those who had relapses under even low levels of stress had significantly higher scores on introversion, neuroticism, and obsessionality. These results are compatible with Eysenck's idea that neuroticism reflects greater emotionality and reactivity. Greater introversion might exacerbate stress reactivity if individuals focus their attention inwardly, or it might reflect reduced access to supportive social relationships to buffer stress. Obsessionality has been hypothesized to interfere with effective social relations (Duggan et al. 1990). Thus, as was found with depressive patients, bipolar patients who display emotional reactivity and indicators of possible reduced social contact were more susceptible to even mild stressors.

It is also noteworthy that the results fail to confirm the hypothesis of Post (1992) and others that relapses without apparent significant stressors are more likely in persons later in their courses of illness. There were no differences between the groups on number of prior episodes (or age at onset), with both stress subgroups reporting multiple prior episodes.

With respect to the high stress groups, those who relapsed were compared with those who did not (who might be considered "resilient" in the face of severe stress). Only two variables distinguished these groups: Those who did not relapse had significantly less family history of psychopathology and significantly lower levels of personality disorder symptoms. It may be that they were "protected" from adverse reactions to high stress by better overall mental health (lower personality disorder symptoms) and by being raised in mentally healthier families. The latter interpretation is consistent with previous research showing that family psychopathology increases offspring risk for disorder not only via genetic but also via psychosocial mechanisms (e.g., Hammen 1991a). In a study on the unipolar outpatients, we found that having higher rates of familial psychopathology predicted worse depressive symptomatology as mediated by early age at onset and higher levels of chronic adversity as well as more episodic stress (Hammen et al. 1992b).

Overall, these findings are exploratory in nature and require replication with large samples. However, they suggest that the variability in responsiveness (relapses) to stressors may have less to do with what Post (1992) has called "neurobiological residues" associated with increased episodes than with psychological factors. Instead, reactivity may have to do with personality variables and "psychosocial residues" that affect an individual's environmental circumstances.

ARE SOME EVENTS MORE "STRESSFUL" THAN OTHERS?

Another reality in the stress disorder research field is that people can undergo objectively dreadful events without necessarily having more than mild and transient symptoms. As noted earlier, the field has reached considerable consensus that it is not the mere occurrence of a negative life event but rather the person's interpretation of the meaning of the event and its significance in the context of its occurrence.

Both psychodynamic theorizing and cognitive-behavioral formulations of depression have hypothesized that individuals may have areas of particular vulnerability—particularly in terms of social relatedness or achievement and autonomy (Arieti and Bemporad 1980; Beck 1983; Blatt et al. 1982). Thus, the experiencing of a social loss or depletion of interpersonal contacts may precipitate a depressive reaction in someone whose sense of self requires social connectedness; it may not affect another person whose self-worth does not depend on relationships. Conversely, someone who derives a sense of efficacy and worth from autonomous achievement might experience depression in the face of a perceived failure. Initially, in a sample of college students, we tested the hypothesis that a specific match between personal vulnerability and type of stressor will produce depression (Hammen et al. 1985). A longitudinal study found support for a link between depressive reactions to stressors whose content matched the area of self-definition, with less depression following stressors whose content did not match. The associations suggested that "sociotropy" and negative interpersonal events are especially predictive of depression.

Subsequently, we extended the hypothesis of a match between specific types of events and individual vulnerability in both unipolar and bipolar outpatients in our longitudinal study. Hammen et al. (1989) administered the Sociotropy-Autonomy Scale (A. Beck et al., unpublished observations, 1983) and classified patients into those with particular emphasis on social connectedness and those with emphasis on achievement and autonomy. Within the first 6 months of follow-up, unipolar patients were more likely to experience onset as well as greater severity of depression if they experienced more events that matched their sociotropy-autonomy status.

With bipolar patients, Hammen et al. (1989) did not find the predicted association between sociotropy-autonomy vulnerability, life events, and symptomatology. However, we reasoned that the 6-month period of follow-up was too brief to permit a full test of the hypothesis. Therefore, we expanded the period of observation to up to 2 years (with a mean ± SD of 18.6 ± 5.9 months) (Hammen et al. 1992a). The sample consisted of 49 bipolar patients; 41 of these showed significant symptom changes during the follow-up, with 25 experiencing major depression, or mania, or mixed states.

Inspection of the timing of events and relapses did not show a significant matching of events and sociotropy-autonomy type. However, there was a significant association with severity of symptomatology. Hierarchical multiple regression analyses were conducted entering sociotropy, interpersonal events, and the interaction of the two terms. (A separate regression was conducted for autonomy, achievement events, and the interaction.) The theory predicts that the interaction of vulnerability and events of that type should significantly predict severity of symptoms. The interaction effect was statistically significant for the prediction of symptoms from sociotropy and interpersonal events (R^2 change = .10, $t = 2.44$, $P < .05$), with the overall equation accounting for 25% of the variance in symptom severity following the events ($F = 5.11$; df = 3,45; $P < .005$). The same analysis of matching autonomy values and achievement events was not significant, however.

Thus, overall there was partial support for the idea that individual vulnerabilities interact with specific negative event content to predict symptoms. The effect was seen for patients' level of vulnerability to social circumstances and the extent of interpersonal events. Also, it did not predict the timing of the onset of symptoms, but it did predict the severity of the symptoms once begun.

Across our various studies—and those of others who have found similar support for the hypotheses in cross-sectional studies—we speculate that the operative mechanism is that events that are interpreted to mean depletion of self-worth and the expectation of inability to replenish the needed supplies will lead to increased symptoms, especially depression. The interpretations of the life events may be distortions or they may be accurate, but we suspect that cognitions associated with self-worth and efficacy are especially critical.

DO PEOPLE CONTRIBUTE TO LIFE EVENT OCCURRENCE?

In both the UCLA Affective Disorders Clinic study and a separate longitudinal study of women with affective disorders and their children conducted by our group (e.g., Hammen 1991a), one of the striking observations that emerged in hundreds of interviews is the extent to which individuals seem to contribute to the actual occurrence of negative events. Stress researchers have long emphasized one direction of causality—from events to symptoms—but I argue that it is essential also to consider the other direction: people contributing to events. Given that affective disorders are recurring and that they take a toll on people around them, such as marital partners and children, I speculate that some individuals have the potential for getting caught up in a vicious cycle of illness and events.

I studied groups of women with unipolar depression, bipolar illness, and chronic medical illness, as well as healthy control women (Hammen 1991b)—all with 8- to 16-year-old children—and followed them longitudinally with methods similar to those of the present study. I found that unipolar women in particular were likely to have high rates of stressors and exceeded all the other groups in events to which they were judged to have at least partly contributed. In specific, they had more interpersonal negative events and, especially, more conflict events (Hammen 1991b). Table 4–1 presents the mean stress ratings by category we examined for the groups under study.

To explore this "stress generation" phenomenon more closely, the types of stressors occurring in the lives of the unipolar and bipolar outpatients in a 1-year period, and their correlates were examined.

The mean objective threat stress totals, defined by independent rating teams, across categories indicated that the unipolar patients had significantly more stress than did the bipolar patients ($t = 2.22$, df = 99, $P < .05$). This appears to be due to differences between the groups on independent event stress only; the groups did not differ significantly on amount of dependent stress (caused at least in part by the individual's behaviors or characteristics), interpersonal event stress, or conflict event stress. Independent events refer to personal illnesses and events that happen to other people. The data suggest that the unipolar patients, more than the bipolar patients, reported medical problems and more negative events happening to their family and friends.

Of particular interest is the extent to which events occurred that were judged to be due at least in part to the person. Figure 4–2 portrays the analysis of total stress for bipolar patients in a 1-year period broken down by proportions of types of events. The data indicate that 63% of bipolar patients' stress was partly or entirely dependent on the person. That is, the majority of stress that these individuals must cope with was due at least in part to their own behaviors or characteristics. (The proportion for the unipolar patients is very similar, 59%.) About half of the dependent stress was primarily interpersonal so that, overall, about 30% of stress was interpersonal. Further, a substantial proportion (73% for unipolar patients and 62% for bipolar patients) of the interpersonal stress specifically concerned conflict with others—lovers and spouses, family members, friends, bosses, and co-workers.

Although there are many aspects of the processes and predictors of stress generation to be explored, my particular interest is in interpersonal stressors and conflict events. I attempted to describe the correlates of interpersonal stress and conflict to get more clues about vulnerability to relapse and aspects of individuals' functioning that might serve as important targets for intervention.

Interpersonal events were divided into nonconflict stress (loss,

Table 4–1. Mean objective stress ratings by group

| Group | Total | Type of event category | | |
		Independent	Dependent	Interpersonal
Unipolar depression	12.7	3.6	8.8	6.3
Bipolar depression	9.1	3.6	5.5	3.2
Medically ill	11.6	6.6	5.1	3.0
Healthy control	7.6	4.4	3.3	2.0

Source. Reprinted with permission from Hammen C: "The Generation of Stress in the Course of Unipolar Depression." *Journal of Abnormal Psychology* 100:555–561, 1991. Copyright 1991, American Psychological Association.

exit, change, entrance events) and conflict stress, and their correlations were computed with three sets of variables: personal psychiatric history factors, personality characteristics, and measures
of attachment-related attitudes. Since unipolar and bipolar patients differed very little on either dependent stress totals or on
these psychiatric and personality variables, the patient groups
were combined to provide a more sensitive test of potentially
important associations. There is no theoretical reason to expect
patient diagnostic differences in the mechanisms by which individuals contribute to their own stressors. Therefore, I explored
the correlates of conflict events in the total group of patients, and
the results are presented in Table 4–2.

Psychiatric History Factors

Degree of conflict stress was modestly but significantly associated with greater extent of psychopathology in first-degree relatives, earlier age at onset, and more frequent previous episodes of
depression ($rs = .20–.32$, $P < .05$). However, none of the background variables were significantly associated with nonconflict
stress.

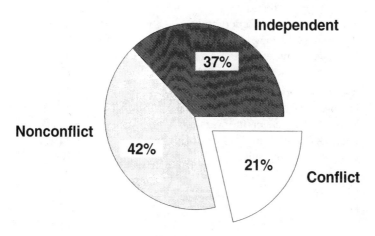

Figure 4–2. Total life stress events: bipolar patients.

Personality Variables

Conflict event stress was significantly but modestly associated with total score on the Personality Disorders Questionnaire, with introversion on the Eysenck Personality Inventory, and with the dependency scale of the Interpersonal Dependency Inventory ($r = .18–.23$, $P < .05$). Neuroticism was unrelated to stress scores. Nonconflict stress was minimally associated with the Personality Disorders Questionnaire total and moderately correlated with the dependency subscale of the Interpersonal Dependency Inventory.

Adult Attachment Attitudes

The associations of interpersonal events and attachment attitudes were tested next. I hypothesized that interpersonal conflict might

Table 4–2. Correlations between conflict event stress and predictor variables: combined unipolar and bipolar patients

Variables	Correlation (r)
Psychiatric background	
Family history of disorder ratings	.20[*]
Age-at-onset ratings	.23[*]
Prior depressive episodes	.32[*]
Prior hospitalizations	.12
Personality score	
Personality Disorders Questionnaire	.23[*]
Eysenck extraversion-introversion	−.18[*]
Eysenck neuroticism	−.13
Interpersonal dependency	.20[*]
Adult Attachment Scale	
Close	−.09
Depend	−.25[**]
Anxiety	.42[*]

[*]$P < .05$. [**]$P < .06$.

be related to underlying insecure attachment based on the theory of Bowlby (1969) and his concept of "working model" cognitions about the self in relation to others that derive from the quality of the early parent-child relationship. The Revised Adult Attachment Scale (Collins and Reed 1990) was administered to a smaller subgroup of patients. This 18-item scale yields three subscales, reflecting the degree to which an individual is comfortable depending on and trusting others (depend), the degree to which he or she is anxious about being abandoned or not being loved (anxiety), and the extent to which he or she is comfortable with closeness and intimacy (close).

The anxiety (abandonment) scale was highly correlated with conflict event stress ($r = .42$, $P < .01$), and comfort and ability to depend on others (depend) was marginally negatively correlated ($r = -.25$, $P = .06$).

Note on Sex Differences

Not only were unipolar and bipolar patients relatively similar in extent of stressors and in scores on their correlates,[1] but also men and women patients were very similar on the variables concerning stressors, psychiatric background, personality, and attachment. However, women reported more conflict stress than did men ($F = 4.23$; df = 1,95; $P < .05$). This overall sex difference was further explored by diagnosis, since previous research had shown that unipolar depressed women experienced significantly more conflict events than did bipolar women (Hammen 1991b). A comparison of unipolar and bipolar women in the present sample revealed that unipolar women reported a significantly higher frequency of conflict events ($P < .05$) and more overall conflict stress ($P = .057$) than did bipolar women. Thus, the uni-

---

[1] Women also reported more depressive episodes than did men ($t = 3.37$, df = 94, $P = .001$). They also scored higher on the Personality Disorders Questionnaire ($t = 2.09$, df = 98, $P < .05$). There were no other significant differences.

polar women seemed to have a somewhat unique pattern of stressors compared with unipolar and bipolar men and women, marked by relatively high levels of conflict with other people.

CONCLUSION

Stress plays an important role in affective disorders. However, there is nothing simple or unidirectional about the stress-symptom association. The relationship between stressors and symptoms is influenced by a wide array of variables, both internal to the person and external in terms of current environmental circumstances. Important design improvements and methodological refinements have made it possible to establish a causal (temporal) association between stressors and depression, and the progression of such work over the past decade has been important. Now, however, attention needs to turn increasingly to individual differences in such processes and to the mediators and mechanisms of the associations.

Conceptual refinements in recent years have emphasized the need to study individual appraisals of stressors in terms of their meaning and implications. Also, the context in which such events occur, including coping resources available to deal with them, greatly affects the meaning and impact of negative events. Recurrent affective disorders have powerful influences on context, potentially creating highly stressful conditions and diminished resources as backgrounds in which episodic stressors occur. Additionally, because of personal experiences and characteristics, as well as in response to recurrent mood disorders and negative events, individuals may contribute to event occurrence. Hence, for many individuals, an unfortunate vicious cycle of disorder-events-disorder may develop. There is much to be learned, for example, about how interpersonal conflict plays a role in recurrent mood disorders.

Although there is relatively little research on stress and bipolar disorders, my longitudinal study of stress in manic-depressive patients adds to the growing appreciation that psychological factors play important roles in the course of the disorder. As the current work shows, some of the same cognitive vulnerabilities and personality characteristics that intensify the impact of stressors for unipolar patients are also seen to affect bipolar patients.

Finally, just as Post (1992) has written of "neurobiological residues" of bipolar episodes that contribute to an endogenous process of episode cycles, it might also be argued that there are "psychological residues" that contribute to recurrence and chronicity in affective disorders. Such processes refer to the psychological sensitivities, increased stress and diminished resources, and the negative impact of the disorders on others—all of which combine to alter both the probability of stress occurrence and the perception that it is unmanageable and depleting, leading to additional symptoms.

The present work has provided preliminary results and speculations about such processes, but considerable work is needed to pursue them. Meanwhile, however, clinical implications are important to explore as well. These findings and those of other investigators strongly support the idea that affective disorders occur in stressful contexts that affect the course of these disorders and the severity of their impact. Such contexts are important targets for therapeutic activity. In addition, individuals' appraisals of situations and their access to and use of supports and resources may be important targets of treatment. It is to be hoped that increased appreciation of the psychosocial context of affective disorders will encourage further vigorous exploration of therapies to supplement the use of biomedical interventions.

REFERENCES

Abramson L, Seligman M, Teasdale J: Learned helplessness in humans: critique and reformulation. J Abnorm Psychol 87:49–74, 1978

Ambelas A: Psychologically stressful events in the precipitation of manic episodes. Br J Psychiatry 135:15–21, 1979

American Psychiatric Association: Diagnostic and Statistical Manual of Mental Disorders, 3rd Edition, Revised. Washington, DC, American Psychiatric Association, 1987

Andrews G, Neilson M, Hunt C, et al: Diagnosis, personality and the long-term outcome of depression. Br J Psychiatry 157:13–18, 1990

Arieti S, Bemporad J: The psychological organization of depression. Am J Psychiatry 137:1360–1365, 1980

Beck A: Cognitive Therapy and the Emotional Disorders. New York, International Universities Press, 1976

Beck A: Cognitive therapy of depression: new perspectives, in Treatment of Depression: Old Controversies and New Approaches. Edited by Clayton PJ, Barrett JE. New York, Raven, 1983, pp 265–290

Bidzinska E: Stress factors in affective diseases. Br J Psychiatry 144:161–166, 1984

Billings A, Cronkite R, Moos R: Social-environmental factors in unipolar depression: comparisons of depressed patients and nondepressed controls. J Abnorm Psychol 93:119–133, 1983

Blatt S, Quinlan D, Chevron E, et al: Dependency and self-criticism: psychological dimensions of depression. J Consult Clin Psychol 50:113–124, 1982

Bowlby J: Attachment and Loss, Vol 1: Attachment. New York, Basic Books, 1969

Brown G, Harris T: Social Origins of Depression. London, Free Press, 1978

Brown G, Bifulco A, Harris T: Life events, vulnerability and onset of depression: some refinements. Br J Psychiatry 150:30–42, 1987

Collins N, Reed S: Adult attachment, working models, and relationship quality in dating couples. J Pers Soc Psychol 58:644–663, 1990

Duggan C, Lee A, Murray R: Does personality predict long-term outcome in depression? Br J Psychiatry 157:19–24, 1990

Dunner D, Patrick V, Fieve R: Life events at the onset of bipolar affective disorder. Am J Psychiatry 136:508–511, 1979

Ellicott A, Hammen C, Gitlin M, et al: Life events and the course of bipolar disorder. Am J Psychiatry 147:1194–1198, 1990

Eysenck H, Eysenck S: Manual of the Eysenck Personality Inventory. San Diego, CA, Educational and Industrial Testing Service, 1978

Glassner B, Haldipur C, Dessauersmith J: Role loss and working-class manic depression. J Nerv Ment Dis 167:530–541, 1979

Glassner B, Haldipur C: Life events and early and late onset of bipolar disorder. Am J Psychiatry 140:215–217, 1983

Gold P, Goodwin F, Chrousos G: Clinical and biochemical manifestations of depression: relation to the neurobiology of stress. N Engl J Med 319:348–353, 1988

Gotlib I, Hammen C: Psychological Aspects of Depression: Toward a Cognitive-Interpersonal Integration. Chichester, England, Wiley, 1992

Hammen C: Stress Runs in Families: The Social Context of Risk and Resilience in Children of Depressed Mothers. New York, Springer-Verlag, 1991a

Hammen C: The generation of stress in the course of unipolar depression. J Abnorm Psychol 100:555–561, 1991b

Hammen C, Marks T, Mayol A, et al: Depressive self-schemas, life stress, and vulnerability to depression. J Abnorm Psychol 94:308–319, 1985

Hammen C, Ellicott A, Gitlin M, et al: Sociotropy/autonomy and vulnerability to specific life events in unipolar and bipolar patients. J Abnorm Psychol 98:154–160, 1989

Hammen C, Ellicott A, Gitlin M: Stressors and sociotropy/autonomy: a longitudinal study of their relationship to the course of bipolar disorder. Cognitive Therapy and Research 16:409–418, 1992a

Hammen C, Davila J, Brown G, et al: Psychiatric history and stress: predictors of severity of unipolar depression. J Abnorm Psychol 101:45–52, 1992b

Harris T, Brown G, Bifulco A: Loss of parent in childhood and adult psychiatric disorder: the role of lack of adequate parental care. Psychol Med 16:641–659, 1987

Harris T, Brown G, Bifulco A: Loss of parent in childhood and adult psychiatric disorder: the role of social class position and premarital pregnancy. Psychol Med 17:163–183, 1987

Harrow M, Goldberg J, Grossman L, et al: Outcome in manic disorders: a naturalistic follow-up study. Arch Gen Psychiatry 47:665–671, 1990

Hirschfeld R, Klerman G, Gough H, et al: A measure of interpersonal dependency. J Pers Assess 41:610–618, 1977

Hirschfeld R, Klerman G, Clayton P, et al: Personality and depression: empirical findings. Arch Gen Psychiatry 40:993–998, 1983

Hirschfeld R, Klerman G, Lavori P, et al: Premorbid personality assessments of first onset of major depression. Arch Gen Psychiatry 46:345–350, 1989

Holahan C, Moos R: Life stressors, personal and social resources, and depression: a 4-year structural model. J Abnorm Psychol 100:31–38, 1991

Hyler S, Rieder R, Williams J, et al: The Personality Disorder Questionnaire: development and preliminary results. Journal of Personality Disorders 2:229–237, 1988

Kennedy S, Thompson R, Stancer H, et al: Life events precipitating mania. Br J Psychiatry 142:398–403, 1983

Klerman G, Weissman M: Increasing rates of depression. JAMA 261:2229–2235, 1989

Lazarus R, Folkman S: Stress, Appraisal, and Coping. New York, Springer-Verlag, 1984

Lazarus R, Folkman S: Transactional theory and research on emotions and coping. European Journal of Personality 1:141–169, 1987

Lewinsohn P, Hoberman H, Rosenbaum M: A prospective study of risk factors for unipolar depression. J Abnorm Psychol 97:251–264, 1988

Lloyd C: Life events and depressive disorders reviewed; II: events as precipitating factors. Arch Gen Psychiatry 37:541–548, 1980

Patrick V, Dunner D, Fieve R: Life events and primary affective illness. Acta Psychiatr Scand 58:48–55, 1978

Post R: Transduction of psychosocial stress into the neurobiology of recurrent affective disorder. Am J Psychiatry 149:999–1010, 1992

Shrout PE, Link B, Dohrenwend B, et al: Characterizing life events as risk factors for depression: the role of fateful loss events. J Abnorm Psychol 98:460–467, 1989

Swindle R, Cronkite R, Moos R: Life stressors, social resources, coping, and the 4-year course of unipolar depression. J Abnorm Psychol 98:468–477, 1989

Thoits P: Dimensions of life events that influence psychological distress: an evaluation and synthesis of the literature, in Psychological Stress: Trends in Theory and Research. Edited by Kaplan HB. New York, Academic Press, 1983, pp 33–103

Wells KB, Stewart A, Hays RD, et al: The functioning and well being of depressed patients: results from the medical outcome study. JAMA 262:914–919, 1989

Chapter 5

The Relationship of Stress to Panic Disorder: Cause or Effect?

Sherry A. Falsetti, Ph.D., Heidi S. Resnick, Ph.D., Bonnie S. Dansky, Ph.D., R. Bruce Lydiard, M.D., Ph.D., and Dean G. Kilpatrick, Ph.D.

P anic disorder (PD) will affect at least one of every 75 people in the United States during their lifetime (Treatment of Panic Disorder 1991). This disorder is characterized by sudden and unexpected discrete periods of intense fear or discomfort associated with at least four of the following symptoms: shortness of breath, choking, rapid heartbeat, chest pain, sweating, dizziness, abdominal distress, hot flashes or chills, numbness or tingling sensations, and a feeling of unreality. In addition, these attacks are often associated with thoughts of "going crazy," losing control, or suffering a heart attack.

Because the symptoms of panic have both physical and cognitive components, this disorder has generated a great deal of attention from biological and cognitive-behavioral researchers. In an effort to understand PD, researchers have examined various factors that may serve to initiate or exacerbate panic. One of the most intriguing new areas under investigation is the relationship of traumatic stress and panic. These two areas of research

This research was partially supported by National Institute of Mental Health Training Grant MH18869-04 and National Institute of Justice Grant 84-IJ-CX-0039.

have not been systematically examined in relation to each other. One reason for this may be that PD as it was defined by DSM-III-R (American Psychiatric Association 1987), required the experience of at least one spontaneous or unexpected panic attack. In other words, there must have been at least one panic attack that did not occur immediately before or at the time of an anxiety-producing event or situation. Thus, attacks that are cued only by specific triggers, such as stressful events, do not meet this criterion.

Those who specialize in treatment and research of reactions to traumatic life events may also be biased against diagnosing panic attacks or PD, instead attributing all physical symptoms to the physiological arousal of posttraumatic stress disorder (PTSD). As a result, few researchers have examined the relationship of PD and traumatic events. In essence, however, many physiological symptoms in PD are identical to those observed in PTSD. Shortness of breath, rapid heart rate, choking, chest pain, dizziness, nausea, feelings of unreality, numbness or tingling sensations, hot flashes or chills, sweating, and trembling or shaking are symptoms of both panic attacks and the physiological arousal of PTSD.

As the anxiety disorders field is evolving, researchers are beginning to question the utility of excluding panic attacks from being diagnosed in the presence of other anxiety disorders. In fact, DSM-IV (American Psychiatric Association 1994) has been revised to list panic attacks prior to the criteria for anxiety disorders, therefore allowing the specification of the absence or presence of panic attacks with other anxiety disorders. This permits the diagnosis of PTSD with panic attacks, thus providing a more accurate clinical description for many patients who have suffered trauma. More importantly, treatment of both PD and PTSD would be more likely to be implemented, thus meeting the needs of patients who have PTSD accompanied by panic attacks. In addition, those with PD and a history of trauma would also be more likely to receive trauma-related treatment if needed. Whether panic attacks associated with PTSD are systematically different or respond differently to treatment is unclear. However, as some have suggested (Ley 1992), use of diagnostic subtypes may provide a better way of assessing the efficacy of more specific treatments. This approach might also result in more treatment outcome research applying cognitive-behavioral techniques that are effective in treating panic attacks in response to the physiological arousal symptoms of PTSD.

Furthermore, as more extensive stressful life event histories are obtained with PD patients, it is becoming evident that many people who are currently diagnosed with PD have experienced traumatic events and that many "spontaneous" attacks may in fact be triggered by subtle cues associated with these stressors. Given the high prevalence rates of traumatic events, which are estimated from 39% to 69% in general population samples (Resnick et al. 1993), it is quite likely that many PD patients are also trauma survivors.

In this chapter, we examine the relationship of panic and life stress, particularly life stress associated with traumatic events. Theories of panic as well as empirical research on the etiology and clinical symptom picture of PD are examined. The literature on the relationship of trauma and panic is reviewed, and biological findings that are relevant to the interrelationship of panic and stress responses are included. In addition, similarities of PD and PTSD, as well as the comorbidity of these disorders, are discussed. There is evidence to suggest that in some cases panic attacks themselves may be the traumatic stressors associated with PTSD (McNally and Lukach 1992). Preliminary results of a study that investigated traumatic events, PD, and PTSD are presented. Finally, a new conceptualization of panic in patients who have experienced traumatic events is introduced.

THEORIES OF PANIC: BIOLOGICAL OR PSYCHOLOGICAL?

Whether biological or cognitive behavioral in orientation, most researchers agree that panic is the experience of fear. It is also generally recognized that fear is normally experienced when danger is present. Most researchers would also readily acknowledge that the experience of fear during a panic attack is often accompanied by a fight-or-flight response, which includes a series of biochemical changes. The fight-or-flight response is a primitive emergency reaction that served humans well when they had to fight or flee predators such as saber-toothed tigers. In present times, such a reaction also occurs when danger is present, for instance, when someone is being attacked physically during a crime. In the case of PD, however, such fear reactions can occur in situations where there is no apparent danger. Thus, researchers often disagree in their understanding of what causes these false alarms of fear in the first place. Specifically, it has been debated whether this condition results from a biological or a psychological malfunction.

Biological Theories of Panic

Most early theories of panic focused on either biological or cognitive dysfunction to explain PD. Biological theorists proposed that there was a neurobiological dysfunction that caused panic. This led to a line of research that attempted to identify a biological marker of panic. Thus far, various pharmacological agents, including lactate, caffeine, isoproterenol, yohimbine, and epinephrine, have all been found to provoke panic, suggesting that there are neurobiological mechanisms associated with the onset of panic attacks (Barlow 1988). In addition, family and twin studies suggest a possible genetic component in PD (Crowe et al. 1983; Harris et al. 1983), although these studies do not support a direct genetic link. Thus, it appears that "vulnerability" to panic, rather than the disorder itself, is inherited.

In sum, there have been many interesting findings, but as of yet no single biological marker of panic has been identified. In fact, Barlow (1988) stated that the only conclusion that can be drawn from psychophysiological and neuroendocrinological studies is that anxious patients appear chronically hyperaroused, hypervigilant, and slow to habituate. According to Barlow, this arousal could be due to genetically determined neurobiological hyperactivity, cognitive helplessness associated with chronic apprehension over future events, or a combination of biological and cognitive factors.

Cognitive-Behavioral Theories of Panic

Early cognitive-behavioral theories of panic proposed that cognitive misattributions in response to somatic symptoms are the cause of panic attacks, such as "I must be having a heart attack" (in response to increased heart rate or chest pain). The initial somatic symptoms themselves are considered normal physiological events, but they occur at inappropriate times (i.e., when no danger is present). According to cognitive theories, it is the catastrophic interpretation of the symptoms that further escalates the symptoms to the level of a panic attack.

A "fear-of-fear" model has also been used to explain the development and maintenance of PD (Jacob and Rapport 1984). This model proposes that situations that are similar to the one in which the initial panic attack took place will cause anticipatory anxiety, setting off another panic attack. It is believed that this conditioning can occur even after a single episode of panic. Consequently, individuals either escape from or avoid feared situations. This results in a lack of extinction, and reinforcement through aversion relief, thus creating a cycle of avoidance. Anticipatory anxiety further increases vigilance, self-monitoring, and self-preoccupation. This can increase awareness of fear-producing external and internal stimuli. Medical conditions are proposed sometimes as the etiology for the first panic response; traumatic events and current conflicts are also implicated. This model invokes learning theory to explain PD but does little to incorporate cognitive components, such as catastrophic thoughts about the attacks.

As is true of most disorders, there is probably not a simple, linear, causal relationship between either biological or cognitive factors and panic. Instead, research suggests that it is probably a combination of biological and cognitive factors that leads to the development of PD. Furthermore, it appears that external factors, particularly stressful life events, may also be important in understanding PD (Barlow 1988).

Biopsychosocial Theory of Panic

Barlow (1988) proposed a model of PD that includes biological, psychological, and social components. According to this model, people who develop PD have a biological vulnerability to overreact to stressful life events that may contribute to the initial panic attack. This vulnerability is considered a biological sensitivity to stress, which may be evidenced by physiological hyperarousal. The reasoning is that if a biological vulnerability is present, then stressors could increase anxiety to such a high level that the physiological symptoms of a panic attack occur. Barlow noted that prior to their first panic attack, people often are in stressful situations that induce intense fear. Yet, the initial attack is a "false alarm" because it occurred when no real physical danger was present. Such spontaneous attacks are considered false alarms because the response that occurs is an overreaction of the system and is not useful.

The false alarm may be the first panic attack to occur but is then followed by anxious anticipation of future panic attacks. This vigilance toward changes in bodily sensations and the interpretations of these changes (e.g., heart attack, "going crazy") are considered the psychological vulnerability component of Barlow's (1988) model. Similar to the fear-of-fear model (Jacob and Rapport 1984), this psychological vulnerability due to increased self-awareness of bodily sensations is a key component of a vicious cycle. Anxious apprehension of further attacks and a focus on somatic cues interact, presumably increasing a fear of normal somatic sensations and the likelihood of future panic attacks. When these bodily sensations actually do occur, the cycle is put in motion. Thoughts about having another attack further increase somatic symptoms, which further increase catastrophic cognitions of danger, which can then escalate to a panic attack.

PANIC AND STRESSFUL LIFE EVENTS

Strong support exists for Barlow's (1988) supposition that people with PD often have a history of stressful life events. Although most patients do not connect their first panic attack to any prior events, if questioned carefully, approximately 80% of patients are able to describe one or more negative life events prior to their first panic attack (Uhde et al. 1985). Typically, stressors such as interpersonal conflict, death of a loved one, major surgery or illness, and other fairly common life events have been assessed.

One of the earliest studies of the association of an anxiety disorder and negative events was conducted by Roth (1959). In this study, 96% of 135 agoraphobic persons were found to have a negative life event prior to developing agoraphobia. More than one-third (37%) reported that a close relative had suddenly developed an illness or had died, and almost one-third (31%) said they had suffered an illness or acute danger prior to the onset of their illness. Another 15% reported domestic stress, and 13% reported panic developing during pregnancy or after childbirth.

Last et al. (1984) assessed negative life event histories of 58 agoraphobic patients. They reported that 81% of these patients had experienced one or more stressful life events prior to the onset of agoraphobia. Negative events that were assessed included interpersonal conflict situations, such as marital-familial conflict (34.5%) and death or illness of a loved one (15.5%). Births, miscarriages, and hysterectomies (29.3%) and drug reactions (12.1%) were also assessed. Finally, major surgery or illness (3.4%), stress at work or school (3.4%), and moving (3.4%) were identified as potential stressors prior to the onset of agoraphobia.

Other studies have also noted the high incidence of life stressors prior to the onset of PD. Doctor (1982) found that separation and loss (31%), relationship problems (30%), and new responsibilities (20%) were commonly reported as stressful events experienced prior to the onset of panic and agoraphobia. In addition, Sheehan et al. (1981) found 91% of their sample had experienced stressful life events. Similarly, Faravelli (1985) and Shafar (1976) also reported high incidences of stressful life events in PD and agoraphobic patients.

It is possible that many of the life events assessed in these studies actually were traumatic stressors, particularly if homicide survivors endorsed items about "sudden death of a relative or friend" or if rape, physical assault, and domestic violence victims endorsed items such as "acute danger" or "interpersonal conflict." However, the prevalence of traumatic events cannot be estimated unless specific assessment of such events is conducted. Without such an investigation of traumatic events experienced by patients with PD, researchers and clinicians cannot attribute panic, or so-called false alarms, to stressful life events.

Unfortunately, except for case studies, traumatic life events such as rape, physical assault, childhood sexual assault, and combat have received very little attention in individuals with PD.

This is surprising given that Roy-Byrne et al. (1986) reported that the quality of stressful events, specifically whether the events were personally threatening or not, was more important than the total number of stressful life events in distinguishing patients with panic attacks from control subjects. Roy-Byrne et al. examined life events in 44 PD patients and 44 control subjects matched for sex and age. Both groups experienced a similar number of life events. However, PD patients reported that the events they experienced were more uncontrollable and undesirable and caused a greater loss of self-esteem compared with control subjects. Unfortunately, Roy-Byrne et al. did not specifically assess events that would be defined as traumatic by DSM-III-R criterion A of PTSD.

Silove (1987) reported several cases of PD, all of whom developed panic attacks after experiencing traumatic events. He described in detail three cases of PD that included a history of sexual abuse. Four other cases that included a history of stressful and/or traumatic events were described briefly. Based on these, Silove proposed that threatening events in childhood predispose individuals to severe anxiety later in life. According to Barlow's (1988) theory, such anxiety would lower the threshold for future panic attacks to occur. The research of Roy-Byrne et al. (1986), Silove, and others would suggest that perhaps it is not necessarily an inborn biological vulnerability that is associated with the initial panic attack but a traumatic event history. In other words, it may not be some undetermined biological factor that brings about the first panic attack for many people but instead a "true alarm" such as physical assault or rape. This experience then may be associated with chronic arousal that could put an individual at risk for subsequent PD. To explore this possibility further, we consider biological and clinical similarities of PD and PTSD.

SIMILARITIES OF PANIC AND PTSD

Traditionally, one must have experienced a traumatic event outside the range of usual human experience and markedly distressing to almost anyone to receive a diagnosis of PTSD. Clearly, stressful events of the most extreme form, such as child sexual abuse, adult rape, and combat, often produce PTSD. What about the association of panic and traumatic events? The diagnosis of panic does not require that one has experienced a traumatic event, as the diagnosis of PTSD does. In fact, as discussed earlier, the diagnosis of PD has typically required the experience of at least one unexpected panic attack. In other words, one panic attack not associated with a stressful event must have been reported. Interestingly, however, we have also noted that people who suffer from PD often do report a history of stressful life events when they are carefully assessed for such events. Thus, initial so-called spontaneous panic attacks may be less common than once thought. Furthermore, it appears that there are both biological and clinical similarities between PD and PTSD. Finally, the limited comorbidity data that do exist suggest that a significant number of people may suffer from both disorders if they have experienced a traumatic event.

Jones and Barlow (1990) noted several similarities between PTSD and PD, including a high proportion of familial psychiatric illness, similar psychophysiological reactions, similar cognitions of unpredictability and uncontrollability, occurrence of negative life events, presence of learned alarms, and anxious apprehension. In addition, Jones and Barlow highlighted similarities in the presentation of panic attacks and flashbacks. Finally, they noted similarities between the emotional numbing in PTSD and the behavioral avoidance found in PD.

Many of the similarities reviewed by Jones and Barlow (1990) are discussed in more detail here, and other possible similarities between PD and PTSD are presented. It is also hypothesized that many people experience panic attacks initiated by a traumatic event but later experience attacks as a conditioned response. Finally, similarities of avoidance are also conceptualized somewhat differently than in the model of Jones and Barlow in that we emphasize the similarities of behavioral avoidance in both disorders rather than compare only the emotional-numbing component of PTSD to avoidance in PD.

Overview of Biological Findings in PD and PTSD

In this section, we briefly review biological similarities and differences between PD and PTSD based on general findings from human studies of family history, neurobiology, sleep patterns, and psychophysiology. Rather than solely reviewing individual studies, we cite reviews of the literature in the areas of panic and PTSD whenever possible.

Family history. As reviewed by Barlow (1988), results of family history studies and particularly studies of monozygotic and dizygotic twins are consistent with the notion that a vulnerability to developing PD is heritable. As noted by Barlow, family history studies in which first-degree relatives of a proband are studied do not control for increased rates of PD due to environment or learning. In twin studies of siblings raised in similar environments with different genetic profiles, the role of genetic and psychosocial factors can be examined more clearly. Results from twin studies indicate significantly higher rates of concordance for PD among monozygotic twins. However, as Barlow pointed out, the fact that the majority of monozygotic twin pairs are discordant for PD suggests an important role for environmental factors in panic etiology. Unfortunately, none of the extant studies include a thorough assessment of traumatic events. Until such assessment is done, it will remain unclear to what extent PD actually differs from PTSD in terms of a predisposing heritable vulnerability related to stress.

Only a few studies have examined family history as a biopsychosocial variable related to PTSD. There are a number of ways that family history of disorder might be associated with PTSD. First, family history of psychopathology might increase risk of exposure to traumatic events. Second, family history of disorder might lead to vulnerability to PTSD after a traumatic event is experienced. This vulnerability could be due to biological predisposition or other factors such as reduced familial social support to assist in posttrauma recovery. Breslau et al. (1991) noted that family history of any psychiatric disorder or substance abuse was associated with increased risk of exposure to traumatic events within a civilian population sample. Results of a study of combat-related PTSD patients (Davidson et al. 1989) and the study by Breslau et al. both indicated higher rates of familial anxiety disorder (not PD specifically) among individuals who had developed PTSD as compared with non-PTSD subjects who had also been exposed to traumatic events.

A major limitation of these two studies is that traumatic event exposure may not have been adequately controlled. For example, Resnick et al. (1993) noted that the rates of rape and sexual assault appeared to be underrepresented within the Breslau et al. (1991) sample, indicating that this type of trauma history was not adequately assessed. Similarly, in the Davidson et al. (1989) study, it was unclear whether degree of combat exposure was equivalent across groups of PTSD and non-PTSD combat veterans. Inadequate control for trauma exposure in these studies could lead to skewed findings regarding the role of family history. Another problem with interpretation of findings noted by Davidson et al. is that high comorbidity of PTSD with other disorders makes the study of family history in PTSD difficult.

There has been one published twin study of PTSD among a sample of 2,092 male monozygotic twin pairs who were either concordant or discordant for service in Southeast Asia or service outside of Southeast Asia (Goldberg et al. 1990). Results were consistent with a significant and primary role for stressor exposure in development of PTSD. Among twin pairs who were discordant for service in Southeast Asia, those who had not served in Southeast Asia had a low rate of PTSD that was comparable with that observed among twins who were concordant for service outside of Southeast Asia. In contrast, members of twin pairs who served in Southeast Asia were two to three times more likely to meet criteria for a presumptive diagnosis of PTSD based on a symptom checklist of DSM-III (American Psychiatric Association 1980) criteria. Probands who had served in Southeast Asia and who had experienced a high degree of combat exposure were nine times more likely to have PTSD than those without service in Southeast Asia. The latter finding further emphasized the importance of assessing not only broad categories of experience but degree and type of critical traumatic incidents.

Study of the role of family history in PTSD development is much more recent than that in the area of panic. Sophisticated direct interview procedures that have been used in the study of PD need to be applied to the study of PTSD. In addition, twin studies and family history studies of PTSD should include careful assessment of all types of potentially traumatic events. Finally, the incorporation of sophisticated trauma assessment within family history studies of PD would allow a more thorough investigation of the role of biological and environmental factors in both PTSD and PD.

Neurobiology. Pitman (1993) reviewed biological studies of neuroregulation in PTSD and noted that findings were consistent with the notion that there is baseline or chronic sympathetic hyperactivity in PTSD. This notion was supported by evidence of increased norepinephrine and epinephrine excretions and adrenergic receptor changes. Results of studies in which trauma-related stimuli were introduced showed increased plasma epinephrine and evidence of a role for the endogenous opioid system in response to stress (Pitman 1993). In terms of neuroregulation abnormalities in PD, there is some evidence for abnormal adrenergic function in PD in studies of the α_2-adrenergic antagonist yohimbine and the α_2-agonist clonidine (E. S. Friedman et al. 1992). The limited data suggest that autonomic dysregulation occurs in both PTSD and PD.

Other studies of both PTSD and panic have included biological challenge tests using sodium lactate or yohimbine and monitoring symptomatic response. Results of studies of panic attacks following lactate infusions among groups of control subjects versus those diagnosed with either PD, major depression, major depression with panic, or social phobia were reviewed by E. S. Friedman et al. (1992). Results indicated that panic attacks were highly specific to groups that had PD and were uncommon within either the control group or the social phobia and depression alone groups. Interestingly, Rainey et al. (1987) reported the occurrence of flashbacks and panic attacks in six of seven male combat veterans following lactate infusion. Pitman (1993) noted that a limitation of this study was that it included only PTSD subjects who also met criteria for PD rather than a broader group. Bremner et al. (1993) controlled for comorbidity by including PTSD patients with and without concurrent PD. Their results indicated a high rate of both panic attacks and flashbacks among PTSD subjects following yohimbine administration. The authors stated that these results suggest a noradrenergic system abnormality in both PTSD and PD. However, as Pitman noted, patients with PD alone do not report flashbacks during panic attacks.

The study of the hypothalamic-pituitary-adrenal (HPA) axis has been of major interest in PTSD research because of its hypothesized role in mediation of the stress response (Yehuda et al. 1991). Results of studies of the HPA axis in PTSD samples indicated low baseline cortisol levels and, contrary to findings for major depression, suppression of cortisol following administration of dexamethasone (Yehuda et al. 1991). In addition, Yehuda et al. indicated that the finding of increased number of glucocorticoid receptors might be consistent with an adaptation of the system to downregulate following chronic stress exposure. As noted by Pitman (1993), findings related to endocrinological functioning in PTSD are primarily consistent with those observed for PD. Specifically, these studies indicated that PD patients respond with a low rate of nonsuppression following dexamethasone similar to that observed in control subjects and dissimilar to that found in depressed patient groups (E. S. Friedman et al. 1992). E. S. Friedman et al. noted that severity of illness and particular symptom profiles may be important factors in dexamethasone response. Given the hypothesized role of the HPA system in the stress response (Yehuda et al. 1991), it is also likely that assessment of major stressor history may be critical in interpretation of these findings. Based on their findings of normal dexamethasone suppression test response among PTSD patients who also met criteria for endogenous major depression, Halbreich et al. (1989) suggested that presence of trauma history may be more critical in understanding dexamethasone suppression test findings than overt symptom profiles.

Pharmacological treatment response.   Research in the pharmacological treatment of PTSD is less developed than it is in PD. There have been few double-blind, controlled studies in PTSD. Descriptive reports have used different assessment approaches, making generalization of findings across reports difficult.

As noted in several reviews (M. J. Friedman 1988; Rosen and Bohon 1990; van der Kolk 1987), different types of pharmacological agents have been reported to be of benefit in treatment of PTSD in open trials and case studies. van der Kolk (1987) summarized the types of drugs that have been studied, including

tricyclic antidepressants, monoamine oxidase inhibitors, benzodiazepines, lithium, carbamazepine, clonidine, β-adrenergic
blockers, and neuroleptics. Of all these agents, there appears to
be least support for the use of neuroleptics (M. J. Friedman 1988).
The other agents may be helpful in decreasing arousal associated
with PTSD (M. J. Friedman 1988; van der Kolk 1987). It has been
suggested that monoamine oxidase inhibitors may be particularly effective in cases where panic symptoms are prominent
(Rosen and Bohon 1990).

Reports of the effectiveness of carbamazepine are of great
interest because demonstrated efficacy would support neurobiological theories suggesting that PTSD symptoms are due to increased neuronal sensitization in association with trauma
exposure (Lipper et al. 1986). Lithium (van der Kolk 1987) and
benzodiazepines (M. J. Friedman 1988) also have been identified
as agents that might have efficacy through similar drug effects.
The limited data for PD indicate a modest antipanic effect for
carbamazepine (Lydiard et al. 1988).

Placebo-controlled, double-blind studies have been conducted
in PTSD with monoamine oxidase inhibitors and tricyclic antidepressants (Davidson et al. 1990). Results indicate some efficacy of
antidepressant medications compared with control conditions in
a subset of studies. As noted by Davidson et al. (1990), other
variables to be assessed include syndrome chronicity and comorbidity, as well as determination of optimal drug dosages and
duration of treatment. Of the agents evaluated in controlled studies, only the tricyclic antidepressants, monoamine oxidase inhibitors, and benzodiazepines have been shown to be unequivocally
effective antipanic agents (Lydiard et al. 1988).

Sleep studies. Data from sleep studies indicate similarities
between PTSD and PD and differences from major depression
(Pitman 1993). For example, in both PTSD and PD, findings do
not indicate presence of reduced rapid eye movement (REM)
latency as has been observed in major depression. However, as
noted by M. J. Friedman (1988), some studies indicate increased
REM latency in PTSD. The presence of disturbed sleep is emphasized among the symptom criteria for PTSD. Disturbed sleep is
categorized as a symptom reflecting general arousal in PTSD,

and the presence of nightmares is included within PTSD diagnostic criteria as a symptom of reexperiencing the traumatic event (American Psychiatric Association 1994).

Ross et al. (1989) suggested that sleep disturbance and disturbances in REM sleep, in particular, might also underlie some other core symptoms of PTSD, such as flashbacks and increased startle response. Although nightmares are not considered a symptom of PD, the phenomenon of nocturnal panic has been studied and is recognized as a significant problem (Craske and Barlow 1989). Interestingly, Craske and Barlow noted that some features of nocturnal panic, such as the autonomic arousal, are similar to night terrors. However, the vivid recall and inability to return to sleep easily differ from night terrors. These same characteristics have been discussed in reference to PTSD nightmares accompanied by autonomic arousal and body movement (Ross et al. 1989). Ross et al. (1989) suggested that this pattern of nightmares might reflect a parasomnia that includes behavioral movement during REM. Interestingly, longer REM latency has been observed in association with nocturnal panic (Mellman and Uhde 1989) similar to results of some studies of PTSD.

Psychophysiology. Results of psychophysiological studies, primarily within combat-exposed samples, indicate that chronic autonomic arousal in PTSD develops posttrauma, as does increased arousal specific to trauma-related cues (Pitman 1993). Pitman noted that the findings in PTSD related to elevated baseline arousal are similar to data on PD patients. However, the elevated arousal to specific cues is similar to that in seen in specific phobias rather than panic.

As summarized by Pitman (1993), there appear to be biological similarities between PTSD and PD in terms of baseline arousal and sleep and neuroendocrine functioning. Major differences include the hypothesized spontaneous onset of PD versus cue-specific arousal in PTSD, the prominence of certain types of intrusive symptoms in PTSD and not PD, and the notion that other conditionable negative emotional reactions beyond just anxiety are likely to be critical in PTSD. Finally, in terms of pharmacological response, Pitman concluded that findings at this time are not helpful regarding questions of nosological classification of PTSD. Future research should include sophisticated procedures for study of pathophysiology in conjunction with sophisticated psychometric assessment measures to identify symptoms of PTSD, panic, and other disorders. As noted by Davidson et al. (1989), it is important to examine groups that have received a "pure" diagnosis as well as groups characterized by comorbidity when studying biological variables. Additionally, future research should incorporate sophisticated assessment of history of traumatic events that may be involved in the stress response across disorders.

Symptoms Common to PTSD and PD

Panic attacks. In terms of symptom presentation, the experience of an alarm reaction accompanied by fear is common to both panic and PTSD. With regard to PTSD, alarm associated with fear is clearly present at the time of the traumatic event. In Barlow's (1988) terminology, this is a "true alarm" because there really was danger present at the time of the event. In addition, recent research indicates that many people experience symptoms of panic attacks during a traumatic event.

One component of the multisite DSM-IV PTSD field trial (Kilpatrick et al. 1992) was the assessment of subjective reactions that occurred during trauma. The major goal of the field trial was to evaluate criterion A for PTSD empirically by studying rates of PTSD symptoms in association with a variety of potentially traumatic events. The sample consisted of 528 adults and adolescents (400 treatment seeking and 128 community) from five geographic locations.

All subjects completed structured interviews and assessments of a comprehensive lifetime history of high-magnitude stressors that included completed rape, other sexual assault, physical assault, other violent crime, homicide death of a family member or close friend, serious accident, natural or man-made disaster, and military combat. In addition, the interview assessed past-year occurrence of events excluded from criterion A in DSM-III-R. Structured PTSD diagnostic interviews were conducted in reference to the lifetime high-magnitude stressor events and the worst, or only, past-year low-magnitude event that may have been experienced. In addition, study participants were asked to report retrospectively their initial emotional and physical reactions at the time they experienced each of these "index" events. A 25-item self-report measure assessed the degree to which the respondent may have experienced each symptom of a panic attack (e.g., shortness of breath, dizziness, fear of going crazy) on a 4-point scale ranging from 1 (not at all) to 4 (extremely). In addition to the 13 items descriptive of panic attacks, several other cognitive and affective responses believed to be important in PTSD development were included (e.g., surprised, helpless, embarrassed, ashamed).

To explore empirically the types of initial reported reactions to events included as high-magnitude DSM-III-R criterion A stressors, a principal-components factor analysis with varimax rotation was conducted on scale responses restricted to the first or only high-magnitude event experienced by respondents (Resnick et al. 1992). The analysis resulted in a five-factor solution that accounted for 61.5% of the variance. Interestingly, the first and largest factor, accounting for 38.5% of the variance, comprised primarily physical symptoms of panic that included dizziness, chest pain, shortness of breath, hot flashes, physical numbing, nausea/gastrointestinal upset, choking, sweating, and fear of going crazy or losing control of emotions or behavior. As can be seen, many of the symptoms of panic were experienced during traumatic events and were important in explaining initial subjective reactions to traumatic events.

Alarm reactions can also occur long after a traumatic event and are part of the symptom picture of PTSD. Based on learning theory models (Keane et al. 1985, 1989) and information-processing theory (Chemtob et al. 1988; Foa et al. 1989), one might expect such alarm panic and stress reactions, as they are responses that were conditioned at the time of the event. Thus any reminders, whether they be external or internal cues, could theoretically trigger arousal or reexperiencing symptoms. Examples of external cues include events such as seeing a story in the newspaper about rape or even the time of day at which the trauma took place. Internal cues such as rapid heartbeat due to exercise could potentially trigger emotions, such as feeling afraid, or thoughts experienced at the time of the event, such as "I'm going to die." Conversely, thoughts that occurred at the time of the event, when reexperienced, could trigger arousal symptoms. These thoughts, whether or not they are attributed to internal or external cues and regardless of whether a conscious connection with the event is made, could further escalate arousal. Such alarm reactions are often evidenced by symptoms of hyperarousal, exaggerated startle response, and physiological reactivity (sweating, rapid heart rate) to reminders of the event(s). Thus, it appears that people who have experienced traumatic events may have panic attacks at the time of the event and, later, as a component of the physiological arousal of PTSD.

It also appears that panic attacks may be common during PTSD flashbacks. Jones and Barlow (1990) noted the similarity of panic attacks and flashbacks. In addition, Mellman and Davis (1985) reported that the most common symptoms accompanying flashbacks in Vietnam veterans were perspiration, tremulousness, palpitations, and dyspnea, all of which are also associated with panic attacks. Horowitz et al. (1980) and Sierles et al. (1983) have also noted panic symptoms in PTSD patients, including increased levels of skin conductance and increased heart rate. These reactions would be considered "learned alarms" because they are conditioned responses to previously neutral stimuli; no real danger is present.

Similarly, PD is accompanied by physiological arousal or alarm reactions, which can include, among other physiological symptoms, sweating, rapid heart rate, and difficulty breathing. In the case of the initial panic attack, Barlow's (1988) model indicates that there may have been stressful events present but that the panic attacks themselves are false alarms because the fight-or-flight response would not be helpful in these situations. In later attacks, the false alarms are in response to the conditioned cues of somatic changes and fears about future attacks. For such attacks, the process is much the same as that of the physiological arousal of PTSD. Reminders of the previous attacks, usually somatic symptoms (e.g., rapid heart rate), cue the panic attack.

Cognitions. In addition to having parallels with regard to physiological arousal symptoms, PTSD and PD may also have similarities in cognitive components and in behavioral avoidance. Recall that panic attacks are often accompanied by thoughts about dying, going crazy, or losing control. Although it is certainly easy to understand that these thoughts may occur in response to the physiological arousal symptoms alone, there may be another explanation in the case of someone with a trauma history. Many people who experience traumatic events believe they may be either injured or killed at the time of the event (Kilpatrick et al. 1987), and they are in fact in a situation that is out of their control. Thus, when the physiological symptoms are present, thoughts of dying or losing control that were experienced at the time of the trauma, as well as feelings of intense fear, may be experienced as part of a conditioned response. In other words, the experience of the cognitive components of panic attacks may be conditioned in much the same way as are the physiological components. Thus it has been hypothesized that an associational network develops in memory after trauma (Foa et al. 1989). This network can be stimulated by physiological, behavioral, cognitive, or affective factors associated with the trauma and can ultimately produce avoidance and escape behavior.

Avoidance. Some other similarities of PD and PTSD worthy of mention are the avoidance symptoms often noted in both disorders. In PTSD these symptoms take the form of avoiding trauma-related thoughts and feelings, as well as avoiding activities and situations that are reminders of the traumatic event. For instance, it is common for a rape victim to avoid watching the news because crimes that remind the victim of the rape may be reported, or to avoid dating for fear of being raped again. There may also be many reminders that are very idiosyncratic that can lead to avoidance. For instance, certain smells, such as the smell of alcohol if the assailant was intoxicated, or places, such as the neighborhood where the rape occurred, can serve as reminders. It is commonly assumed that people with PTSD are avoidant because to be reminded of a trauma is psychologically very painful and distressing. Although this is undoubtedly very true, it should also be noted that reminders often trigger the physiological reactivity of PTSD, which can include sweaty palms, increased heart rate, shortness of breath, and other arousal symptoms that also happen to be the symptoms of panic attacks and are themselves very distressing.

In the case of PD, avoidance is often present as agoraphobia. To meet the diagnostic criteria for PD with agoraphobia, the criteria for PD first must be met. In addition, fear of being in places or situations from which escape might be difficult or in which help might not be available in the event of a panic attack must also be present. During such situations, intense anxiety is often experienced, and the person typically avoids these situations (DSM-IV criteria). Again, the similarity between the avoidance noted in PTSD and PD is very striking and in many cases may even be motivated by similar circumstances, namely fear of intense physiological arousal and cognitions of danger—symptoms that have also been identified with panic attacks. In sum, it appears there are many clinical similarities among the symptoms of PD and PTSD.

So far it has been demonstrated that there are many etiological, biological, and clinical similarities of PTSD and PD. Given these similarities, an investigation of the comorbidity of these disorders is also important. First, the little comorbidity research that does exist is reviewed. This is followed by a presentation of preliminary results of a study conducted at the National Crime Victims Research and Treatment Center at the Medical University of South Carolina in Charleston, which investigated traumatic events and the comorbidity of PTSD and panic.

COMORBIDITY OF PD AND PTSD

In an article on comorbidity, Kendall and Clarkin (1992) stated that the "study of comorbidity is the premier challenge facing mental health professionals in the 1990s" (p. 833). Indeed, untangling the threads of two or more disorders that may be intertwined on so many levels is certainly a challenge. The study of comorbidity of mental disorders is fairly new, and there is still much work ahead. Yet, such research may be critical for effective diagnosis and treatment of many disorders. This may be particularly true in the area of PD and PTSD, given some of the biological and psychological similarities, as well as the high prevalence of traumatic event histories, often present in patients with both disorders.

Most comorbidity research on PD has been in relation to disorders other than PTSD. For instance, in an article that specifically focused on comorbidity among anxiety disorders, Brown and Barlow (1992) reported comorbidity rates of PD in association with social phobia, generalized anxiety disorder, obsessive-compulsive disorder, simple phobia, major depressive episode, and dysthymia. Although the results were certainly noteworthy, they failed to report comorbidity rates for PTSD and PD.

Studies that have investigated comorbidity of PD and PTSD have reported a substantial co-occurrence of the two disorders. For instance, in examining the effects of wartime stressors in Vietnam veterans who were psychiatric inpatients, Breslau and Davis (1987) reported that 77% of their sample met DSM-III criteria for PTSD, and 32% met criteria for PD. Although they reported that the impact of participation in atrocities was not significant in predicting PD, they found that the number of combat stressors was a significant predictor of PD and was similar in magnitude to the significance of this variable in predicting PTSD.

Similarly, Green et al. (1990) examined risk factors for PTSD and other diagnoses in a sample of Vietnam veterans. Unlike the Breslau and Davis (1987) study, however, this study included subjects who were not seeking treatment (two-thirds of the sample), as well as treatment seekers. Of this sample, 29% met diagnostic criteria for PTSD, 7% met criteria for PD, and 5% met criteria for both PTSD and PD. In addition, the results of the regression analyses for the prediction of these disorders by premilitary, military, and postmilitary variables were very similar to each other. War stressor factors were highly predictive of PTSD and were also strongly predictive of PD. Although PTSD was the only diagnosis predicted by life threat, PD was predicted by dangerous assignment activities, which held the potential threat of capture or sudden death, and included repeated and prolonged arousal, again highlighting the similarities between panic and PTSD.

Taking a somewhat different perspective, Davidson et al. (1990) compared symptoms and comorbidity patterns between 19 World War II and 25 Vietnam War veterans with PTSD. Overall, Vietnam veterans were found to exhibit more severe PTSD than World War II veterans. The most frequent comorbid diagnoses were PTSD and generalized anxiety disorder, followed by PTSD and PD. In terms of panic attacks, there were no significant differences in the number of veterans who reported attacks based on whether they had been in the Vietnam War or World War II. In both samples, approximately 50% of the veterans reported panic attacks. However, there were differences between the groups in meeting the full diagnostic criteria for PD. In the World War II sample, 10.5% met the criteria, whereas in the Vietnam veteran group, 44% had a lifetime diagnosis of PD. With regard to time of onset, in only one case did a diagnosis of PD precede a diagnosis of PTSD. In all other cases, PD either developed the same year or anywhere from 1 to 18 years later. Finally, Rainey et al. (1990) also noted relationships between PTSD and PD associated with combat. They reported on rates of comorbid PTSD and PD in Vietnam veterans with chronic PTSD. Of 40 subjects with chronic PTSD, 24 (60%) also met criteria for current PD.

In all of the research reviewed thus far, it has been presumed that the co-occurrence of PD and PTSD may be related to traumatic stressors that could potentially predispose one to the development of these disorders. However, there has been at least one study that investigated panic attacks as traumatic stressors. McNally and Lukach (1992) examined 30 people with PD. Subjects were asked to identify their most frightening panic attacks and then were interviewed using the Structured Clinical Interview for DSM-III-R (SCID; Spitzer et al. 1990) to assess PTSD symptomatology in response to those panic attacks. McNally and Lukach reported that 17% of the subjects met the criteria for lifetime PTSD, and 7% met the criteria for current PTSD with a panic attack as their identified traumatic event.

Although patients with a history of trauma were presumably ruled out, it was not clear how effectively this was done. As previously noted, without a very careful traumatic events assessment, many people with a history of trauma may not have been detected and ruled out. Thus, if some people with such a history were included, it is possible that either the panic attacks they experienced were a result of chronic hyperarousal, which would leave them more susceptible to panic attacks, or the panic attacks may have been associated with some unidentified trauma-related cues. It also would have been informative to know what percentage of the potential panic sample did, in fact, have to be ruled out due to trauma history. Given the high base rates in the general population alone, it would seem likely that a good number of people in this sample may have experienced traumatic events other than their panic attacks.

All of the research reviewed thus far is supportive of a relationship among stressful events, PTSD, and PD. There are two major shortcomings, however. First, few if any researchers investigating the relationship among these variables have conducted thorough trauma assessment histories. Second, the comorbidity research on PD and PTSD has largely investigated combat veterans and does not address comorbidity within other trauma populations and therefore may not be generalizable. In an effort to address these issues, some preliminary results from a study that included thorough trauma assessments with a representative community sample are presented. Data on victim characteristics, trauma prevalence rates, and associated rates of PTSD in this sample are described in detail elsewhere (Kilpatrick et al. 1987). We briefly summarize demographic characteristics and trauma prevalence data, but focus primarily on a detailed examination of crime characteristics associated with PD and comorbidity of PD and PTSD.

TRAUMA, PANIC, AND PTSD: PRELIMINARY REPORT

Methodology

Respondents.   A total of 391 female adults participated in the current study. These women were a subset of a representative community sample of 1,467 in Charleston, South Carolina. The mean age for the respondents was 39.8 years, with a range of 18–83. The racial makeup of the sample was (non-Hispanic) Caucasian (72.9%) or (non-Hispanic) African-American (26.6%), and less than 1% of the sample consisted of other racial-ethnic groups. A majority of the respondents were married (65.0%); 14.8% had never been married, 10% were widowed, and 10.3% were divorced or separated.

More than one-half of the respondents were employed full- or part-time (77.3%), and about one-fourth reported that they were homemakers (26.1%). The modal family income range for the sample was $7,500 or less (11.5%), $7,501–$15,000 (15.1%), $15,001–$25,000 (26.1%), $25,001–$35,000 (21.5%), $35,001–$50,000 (12.8%), and $50,001 or more (10%). Finally, with respect to educational background, more than one-half of the respondents had graduated from high school (53.5%). An additional 9.7% received postgraduate education, 18.2% were college graduates, 4.9% had received vocational or technical training following high school, and 13.8% never completed high school.

Assessment instruments. Three structured interviews were used: the Incident Report Interview (Kilpatrick et al. 1987), Diagnostic Interview Schedule (DIS; Robins et al. 1981), and a slightly modified version of the SCID (SCID-PTSD). The Incident Report Interview, designed to evaluate respondents' victimization history, consisted of behaviorally specific probes to detect eight types of major crimes, including rape, aggravated assault, robbery, and burglary (for further details, see Kilpatrick et al. 1989; Resnick et al. 1992). The DIS and SCID-PTSD interviews, which have been shown to be reliable instruments for assigning psychiatric diagnoses (Robins et al. 1981; Spitzer et al. 1987), were utilized to assess PD and PTSD.

The DIS is a structured interview schedule that was designed to be administered by lay interviewers to determine both lifetime and current psychiatric disorders, including PD, major depression, agoraphobia, social phobia, simple phobia, and obsessive-compulsive disorder. Since at the inception of the current investigation the DIS did not include a set of questions to evaluate PTSD, assessment questions were developed based on the criteria for PTSD outlined in DSM-III. This instrument closely resembles the PTSD module of the SCID. The PTSD interview was administered to all respondents who reported some type of criminal victimization on the Incident Report Interview.

Respondents were classified as having current PTSD if their

symptoms were current at the time of the interview. Lifetime PTSD encompassed all respondents who reported symptoms that met the criteria for PTSD at some point during their lives. Respondents who reported symptoms of panic were classified as having "panic attacks"; those who reported symptoms that met the full criteria for PD were also classified in the PD group.

Procedures. The Incident Report Interview was first administered to the respondents by female research assistants; the DIS and SCID-PTSD interviews were administered by clinical psychologists, psychology interns, or social workers. The DIS was administered to all respondents, and the interviewers were blind to the respondents' victimization history. Only during the PTSD module of the SCID were the clinical interviewers made aware of the participants' victimization history. This procedure was necessary, since only respondents who reported an incident of criminal victimization completed the PTSD interview, and the PTSD symptom criteria were linked to the previously assessed crime incidents.

For respondents in the crime victim group, the time frame for the occurrence of any non-PTSD psychiatric disorder was assessed in relation to each victimization such that respondents who met lifetime criteria for the non-PTSD disorder were asked whether the disorder was present before, after, or both before and after their first exposure to a traumatic crime. In addition, lifetime PTSD was evaluated in reference to respondents' first or only crime exposure or their self-identified worst crime exposure (if more than one crime was reported).

Preliminary Results

Of the sample of 391 respondents, 295 crime victims were identified. The following crimes were reported by the respondents: sexual assault 52.9%, aggravated assault 9.7%, robbery 5.6%, and burglary 45.3% (some victims reported more than one crime). The sample prevalence rates for lifetime and current PTSD using DSM-III criteria were 21% and 5.6%, respectively. Furthermore, 7.9% of the sample reported panic attacks, and 4.6% met full criteria for PD.

The prevalence of crime victimization among respondents with PD was assessed by chi-square analyses. The overall rate of crime victimization among PD respondents was 94.4%; only one participant with PD did not report a victimization (Table 5–1). A similarly high rate of victimization was found among respondents with panic attacks (93.5%). When respondents with PD were compared with respondents not reporting panic symptoms (non-PD), a significantly higher proportion of respondents with PD (27.8%) reported an aggravated assault than respondents in the non-PD group (8.8%; χ^2 = 7.01, df = 1, P < .01). There were no other significant differences between respondents in the PD and non-PD groups for type of victimization. However, when all respondents with panic attacks were assessed, this group had a significantly higher proportion of crime victimization in general (93.5%) than respondents without panic attacks (73.9%; χ^2 = 5.96, df = 1, P < .05).

Comorbidity of PD and PTSD was also examined. The prevalence of lifetime PTSD among respondents diagnosed with PD was 44.4%, and current PTSD was observed in 22.2% of PD respondents (Table 5–1). Chi-square analyses comparing respondents with PD with those in the non-PD group yielded significant results for lifetime and current PTSD. More specifically, the prevalence of lifetime PTSD among respondents with PD (44.4%) was significantly higher than among respondents in the non-PD group (19.8%; χ^2 = 6.27, df = 1, P < .05). A parallel pattern of results was obtained for current PTSD in that a significantly higher proportion of respondents with PD (22.2%) as compared with non-PD respondents (4.8%) reported current symptoms of PTSD (χ^2 = 9.79, df = 1, P < .01).

Discussion

The results of this study indicate an extremely high prevalence of criminal victimization among respondents with PD. The comorbidity rates of PTSD and PD were also significant and were somewhat higher than comorbidity rates reported for combat veterans, with the exception of those reported by Davidson et al. (1990), who found that 44% of their Vietnam veteran group met the criteria for lifetime PD. The results of this study are certainly compelling and provide further support for our hypothesis about associations among stressful events, PD, and PTSD.

TOWARD A NEW CONCEPTUALIZATION OF STRESS AND PANIC

Based on the empirical research presented here, information processing theory (Chemtob et al. 1988; Foa et al. 1989), and Barlow's (1988) model of PD, a heuristic model of panic for people who have experienced traumatic stress is presented. This model incorporates Barlow's concept of alarms but questions whether biological or psychological vulnerability must be present for panic to

Table 5–1. Percentages of victimization and posttraumatic stress disorder (PTSD) among participants with panic disorder (PD)

	Lifetime PD (N = 18)		Panic attacks (N = 31)	
	%	n	%	n
Nonvictim	5.6	1	6.5	2
Crime victim	94.4	17	93.5[*]	29
Any sexual assault	55.6	10	64.5	20
Aggravated assault	27.8[**]	5	16.1	5
Robbery	5.6	1	6.5	2
Burglary	61.1	11	61.3	19
Completed rape	27.8	5	35.5	11
Sexual molestation	16.7	3	19.4	6
Other sexual assault	16.7	3	25.8	8
Lifetime PTSD	44.4[*]	8	48.4	15
Current PTSD	22.2[**]	4	25.8	8

[*]$P < .05.$ [**]$P < .01.$

develop in individuals who have experienced traumatic events that would be distressing to almost anyone. Another difference between the model that is presented here and Barlow's model of panic is that the occurrence of a traumatic event may lead to the avoidance symptoms of PTSD, whereas in the absence of trauma, avoidance symptoms associated with panic are considered ago-raphobic symptoms. Although the labels for the avoidance are different for each disorder, the avoidance in both appears to be an attempt to reduce the probability of experiencing distressful psychological and physiological reactions. Our model of the de-velopment of panic in individuals who have experienced trau-matic events is presented in Figure 5–1.

We propose that it may not be some undetermined biological factor alone that brings about the first panic attack for many people, but instead a true alarm in response to physical assault or rape. Given this, both external and internal stimuli associated with a traumatic event could be conditioned and could later trigger "learned alarms." Examples of external cues include places, situations, objects, smells, and sounds associated with the trauma. Internal cues include emotions, the physiological arousal experienced during traumatic events, and cognitions about dying or going crazy, which may have been cognitions experienced at the time of an event.

Therefore, actual external cues associated with events, internal cues such as physiological arousal that were experienced at the time of the event, or emotions experienced during the time of traumatic events (fear, disgust) together form an information-processing network of which any component could potentially trigger other components of the network and hence future panic attacks. Such attacks may seem to be out of the blue, as many of these cues may not be perceived as directly connected to an event. In addition, the chronic hyperarousal and hypervigilance, which Barlow (1988) described as some of the most consistent symptoms in PD patients, may be associated with traumatic events. A psychological vulnerability as described by Barlow may be present but is not viewed as necessary to develop either a conditioned emotional response or avoidance symptoms. Finally, the avoidance symptoms are hypothesized to strengthen further the associational network of conditioned cues and responses

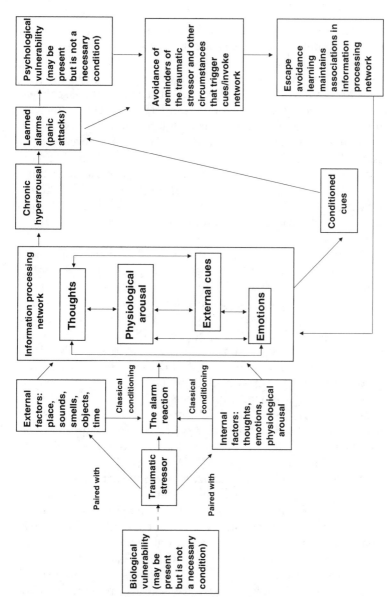

Figure 5–1. A proposed model of panic disorder associated with traumatic stressors.

through escape-avoidance learning and lack of extinction, thereby maintaining a cycle of chronic hyperarousal and panic attacks.

Thus, it appears not only that panic may develop directly from a past traumatic experience but that such an experience can lead to the chronic hyperarousal noted in PTSD, which can increase future vulnerability to panic through kindling or decreasing the amount of further arousal needed to reach the threshold for panic. Therefore, a previous traumatic stressor, although perhaps not readily identified by the patient in connection with panic attacks, may have increased arousal levels to a point where it may then take only relatively minor stressors to reach the threshold for the physiological symptoms of a panic attack to occur (see Figure 5–2).

Because there may be no actual physical danger at the time of these future attacks, it is also possible that when such physiological symptoms do occur, the individual becomes frightened and focuses on the arousal symptoms, thinking he or she is having a heart attack, going crazy, or dying (Barlow 1988). In fact, evidence suggests that many patients with PD demonstrate a specific hypervigilance to signs of threat (Mathews and MacLeod 1986) and that many patients with PD are excessively preoccupied with fears of physical danger (Hibbert 1984). If many of these people did indeed experience what they perceived to be life-threatening events or PTSD criterion A events, these responses would not be unusual. Again, these are symptoms commonly reported by people who have experienced traumatic events and are suffering from PTSD.

As noted, such a conceptualization is consistent not only with learning theory but also with information-processing theory, which has been applied to PTSD. Foa et al. (1989) proposed an information-processing theory based on Lang's model (1977). Foa et al.'s model postulates that information about traumatic events is stored in a fear network, which is made up of stimuli, responses, and the meaning of the stimulus and response elements. This network is considered a sort of "program" that creates the avoidance behavior of PTSD if activated. The network can be activated by any part of the fear network. Thus, cognitions that were present at the time of traumatic events, such as "I have no control over what is going to happen to me," could later in a completely different setting induce feelings of fear or physiological arousal symptoms. Similarly, feelings of fear or physiological arousal symptoms could facilitate thoughts about being unable to escape or thoughts about death that may have been present at the time of the traumatic event. In addition, Litz and Keane (1989) found that anxious subjects have an attentional bias toward threat cues. If such a theory is applied to the understanding of panic in people with a traumatic event history, then it would be expected that physiological cues would be considered part of that fear network, and vigilance toward such cues would further increase the likelihood of future panic attacks.

It should be cautioned that we are in no way attempting to explain all cases of PD. It is likely that there is heterogeneity within PD. Thus, for a subset of those with PD, experiences such as physical illness (e.g., heart problems) or other less severe stressors may interact with some vulnerability to lead to development of PD. In other cases, as hypothesized for PTSD, it is possi-

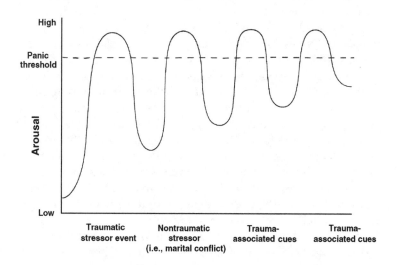

Figure 5–2. The development of panic in relation to arousal levels.

ble that PD may occur in those without prior vulnerability following exposure to true alarm.

Based on the empirical data presented, it appears that thorough assessment of trauma history may aid our progress in understanding the etiology of panic. As noted, the rates of trauma even in general population samples are astounding. One can only assume that they are even higher in patient populations. Because of this, trauma histories should be carefully assessed in all patients coming in for treatment. It should also be noted that how patients are asked about trauma histories greatly affects what is reported. To assess trauma thoroughly, questions must be behaviorally specific. For instance, much more accurate information is likely to be obtained from asking, "Has anyone ever used pressure, coercion, or nonphysical threats to have sexual contact with your sexual organs or to make you have sexual contact with their sexual organs?" than from asking, "Have you ever been raped?" In fact, the lower prevalence rates for trauma reported in some studies have been attributed to the failure to conduct behaviorally specific trauma assessments (Resnick et al. 1993).

Finally, the implications for treatment of patients with PTSD, with PD, and with both disorders must be considered. As the anxiety disorder field progresses and the similarities of panic attacks and physiological arousal of PTSD become recognized, cognitive-behavioral treatments, such as that developed by Barlow and Craske (1988), that have been used in treating PD should be investigated for the treatment of the arousal symptoms of PTSD. If the arousal symptoms were to become less aversive and frightening after such treatment, other PTSD treatments, such as imaginal exposure to the trauma, may be more palatable to both clinicians and patients. With regard to PD, if a trauma history is identified, the panic may be related to trauma cues. Having this information would aid in planning treatment for these patients that could address both their panic symptoms and their trauma histories. Such information may in itself be therapeutic for patients in providing some understanding of their symptoms and in dispelling fears of physical illnesses, such as heart attacks. In addition, PTSD should also be assessed in those patients who are reporting panic and a history of trauma. It is only through careful assessment that effective treatment and future progress in our understanding of the role of stress in psychological disorders can be achieved.

REFERENCES

American Psychiatric Association: Diagnostic and Statistical Manual of Mental Disorders, 3rd Edition. Washington, DC, American Psychiatric Association, 1980

American Psychiatric Association: Diagnostic and Statistical Manual of Mental Disorders, 3rd Edition, Revised. Washington, DC, American Psychiatric Association, 1987

American Psychiatric Association: Diagnostic and Statistical Manual of Mental Disorders, 4th Edition. Washington, DC, American Psychiatric Association, 1994

Barlow DH: Anxiety and Its Disorders. New York, Guilford, 1988

Barlow DH, Craske MG: Mastery of Your Anxiety and Panic. Albany, NY, Center for Stress and Anxiety Disorders, 1988

Bremner JD, Davis M, Southwick SM, et al: Neurobiology of posttraumatic stress disorder, in American Psychiatric Press Review of Psychiatry, Vol 12. Edited by Oldham JM, Riba MC, Tasman A. Washington, DC, American Psychiatric Press, 1993, pp 183–204

Breslau N, Davis GC: Posttraumatic stress disorder: the etiologic specificity of wartime stressors. Am J Psychiatry 144:578–583, 1987

Breslau N, Davis GC, Andreski P, et al: Traumatic events and posttraumatic stress disorder in an urban population of young adults. Arch Gen Psychiatry 48:216–222, 1991

Brown TA, Barlow DH: Comorbidity among anxiety disorders: implications for treatment and DSM-IV. J Consult Clin Psychol 60:835–844, 1992

Chemtob C, Roitblat HL, Hamada RS, et al: A cognitive action theory of post-traumatic stress disorder. Journal of Anxiety Disorders 2:253–275, 1988

Craske MG, Barlow DH: Nocturnal panic. J Nerv Ment Dis 177:160–167, 1989

Crowe RR, Noyes R, Pauls DL, et al: A family study of panic disorder. Arch Gen Psychiatry 40:1065–1069, 1983

Davidson J, Smith R, Kudler H: Familial psychiatric illness in chronic posttraumatic stress disorder. Compr Psychiatry 30:339–345, 1989

Davidson J, Kudler HS, Saunders WB, et al: Symptom and comorbidity patterns in World War II and Vietnam veterans with posttraumatic stress disorder. Compr Psychiatry 31:162–170, 1990

Doctor RM: Major results of a large-scale pretreatment survey of agoraphobics, in Phobia: A Comprehensive Summary of Modern Treatments. Edited by Dupont RL. New York, Brunner/Mazel, 1982, pp 203–214

Faravelli C: Life events preceding the onset of panic disorder. J Affect Disord 9:103–105, 1985

Foa EB, Steketee G, Olasov-Rothbaum B: Behavioral/cognitive conceptualizations of post-traumatic stress disorder. Behavior Therapy 20:155–176, 1989

Friedman ES, Clark DB, Gershon S: Stress, anxiety, and depression: review of biological, diagnostic, and nosologic issues. Journal of Anxiety Disorders 6:337–363, 1992

Friedman MJ: Toward rational pharmacotherapy for posttraumatic stress disorder: an interim report. Am J Psychiatry 145:281–285, 1988

Goldberg J, True WR, Eisen SA, et al: A twin study of the effects of the Vietnam war on posttraumatic stress disorder. JAMA 263:1227–1232, 1990

Green BL, Grace MC, Lindy JD, et al: Risk factors for PTSD and other diagnoses in a general sample of Vietnam veterans. Am J Psychiatry 147:729–733, 1990

Halbreich U, Olympia J, Carson S, et al: Hypothalamo-pituitary-adrenal activity in endogenously depressed post-traumatic stress disorder patients. Psychoendocrinology 14:365–370, 1989

Harris EL, Noyes R, Crowe RR, et al: Family study of agoraphobia. Arch Gen Psychiatry 40:1061–1064, 1983

Hibbert GA: Ideational components of anxiety: Their origin and content. Br J Psychiatry 144:618–624, 1984

Horowitz MJ, Wilner N, Kaltrieder N, et al: Signs and symptoms of post-traumatic stress disorder. Arch Gen Psychiatry 37:85–92, 1980

Jacob RG, Rapport MD: Panic disorder: medical and psychological parameters, in Behavioral Theories and Treatment of Anxiety. Edited by Turner SM. New York, Plenum, 1984, pp 187–237

Jones JC, Barlow DH: The etiology of posttraumatic stress disorder. Clinical Psychology Review 10:299–328, 1990

Keane TM, Zimering RT, Caddell JM: A behavioral formulation of posttraumatic stress disorder in Vietnam veterans. The Behavior Therapist 8:9–12, 1985

Keane TM, Fairbank JA, Caddell JM, et al: Implosive (flooding) therapy reduces symptoms of PTSD in Vietnam combat veterans. Behavior Therapy 20:245–260, 1989

Kendall PC, Clarkin JF: Introduction to special section: comorbidity and treatment implications. J Consult Clin Psychol 60:833–834, 1992

Kilpatrick DG, Saunders BE, Veronen LJ, et al: Criminal victimization: lifetime prevalence, reporting to police, and psychological impact. Crime and Delinquency 33:479–489, 1987

Kilpatrick DG, Saunders BE, Amick-McMullan A, et al: Victim and crime factors associated with the development of crime-related post-traumatic stress disorder. Behavior Therapy 20:199–214, 1989

Kilpatrick DG, Resnick HS, Freedy JR, et al: Report of Findings from the DSM-IV PTSD Field Trial Emphasis on Criterion A and Overall PTSD Diagnosis (final report submitted to the National Institute of Mental Heath, Grant No 1 PO1 MH47200-01). Bethesda, MD, National Institute of Mental Health, 1992

Last CG, Barlow DH, O'Brien GT: Precipitants of agoraphobia: Role of stressful life events. Psychol Rep 54:567–570, 1984

Lang PJ: Imagery in therapy: an information processing analysis of fear. Behavior Therapy 8:862–886, 1977

Ley R: Hyperventilatory, anticipatory, and cognitive panic attacks. Paper presented at the annual meeting of the Association for the Advancement of Behavior Therapy, Boston, MA, November 1992

Lipper S, Davidson JRT, Grady TA, et al: Preliminary study of carbamazepine in post-traumatic stress disorder. Psychosomatics 27:849–854, 1986

Lizt BT, Keane TM: Information processing in anxiety disorders: application to the understanding of post-traumatic stress disorder. Clinical Psychology Review 9:243–257, 1989

Lydiard RB, Roy-Byrne PD, Ballenger JC: Recent advances in the psychopharmacological treatment of anxiety disorders. Hosp Community Psychiatry 39:1157–1165, 1988

Mathews AM, MacLeod C: Discrimination of threat cues without awareness in anxiety states. J Abnorm Psychol 95:131–138, 1986

McNally RJ, Lukach BM: Are panic attacks traumatic stressors? Am J Psychiatry 149:824–826, 1992

Mellman TA, Davis GC: Combat related flashbacks in posttraumatic stress disorder: phenomenology and similarity to panic attacks. J Clin Psychiatry 46:379–382, 1985

Mellman TA, Uhde TW: Electroencephalographic sleep in panic disorder: a focus on sleep related panic attacks. Arch Gen Psychiatry 46:178–184, 1989

Pitman R: Biological findings in posttraumatic stress disorder, in Post-traumatic Stress Disorder: DSM-IV and Beyond. Edited by Davidson JRT, Foa EB. Washington, DC, American Psychiatric Press, 1993, pp 173–189

Rainey JM, Aleem A, Ortiz A, et al: A laboratory procedure for the induction of flashbacks. Am J Psychiatry 144:1317–1319, 1987

Rainey JM, Manov G, Aleem A, et al: Relationships between PTSD and panic disorder: concurrent psychiatric illness, effects of lactate infusions, and erythrocyte lactate production, in Clinical Aspects of Panic Disorder. Edited by Ballenger JC. New York, Wiley, 1990, pp 47–54

Resnick HS, Kilpatrick DG, Dansky BS, et al: Emotional and physiological responses during a variety of traumatic events. Paper presented at the annual meeting of the Association for the Advancement of Behavior Therapy, Boston, MA, November 1992

Resnick HS, Kilpatrick DG, Dansky BS, et al: Prevalence of civilian trauma and posttraumatic stress disorder in a representative national sample of women. J Consult Clin Psychol 61:984–991, 1993

Robins LN, Helzer JE, Croughan J, et al: National Institute of Mental Health Diagnostic Interview Schedule: Its History, Characteristics, and Validity. Arch Gen Psychiatry 38:381–389, 1981

Rosen J, Bohon S: Posttraumatic stress disorder: pharmacotherapy, in Handbook of Comparative Treatments for Adult Disorders. Edited by Bellack AS, Hersen M. New York, Wiley, 1990, pp 316–326

Ross RJ, Ball WA, Sullivan KA, et al: Sleep disturbance as the hallmark of posttraumatic stress disorder. Am J Psychiatry 146:697–707, 1989

Roth M: The phobic anxiety-depersonalization syndrome. Proceedings of the Royal Society of Medicine 52:587–596, 1959

Roy-Byrne PP, Geraci M, Uhde TW: Life events and the onset of panic disorder. Am J Psychiatry 143:1424–1427, 1986

Shafar S: Aspects of phobic illness: a study of 90 personal cases. Br J Med Psychol 49:221–236, 1976

Sheehan DV, Sheehan KE, Minichiello WE: Age of onset of phobic disorders: a reevaluation. Compr Psychiatry 22:544–553, 1981

Sierles FS, Chen JJ, McFarland RE, et al: Post-traumatic stress disorder and concurrent psychiatric illness: a preliminary report. Am J Psychiatry 140:177–179, 1983

Silove D: Severe threat in the genesis of panic disorder. Aust N Z J Psychiatry 21:592–600, 1987

Spitzer RL, Williams JBW, Gibbon M: Structured Clinical Interview for DSM-III-R: Nonpatient Version (SCID-NP-V). New York, New York State Psychiatric Institute, 1987

Spitzer RL, Williams JBW, Gibbon M, et al: Structured Clinical Interview for DSM-III-R. Washington, DC, American Psychiatric Press, 1990

Treatment of Panic Disorder: NIH Consensus Development Conference Consensus Statement, September 25–27, 1991

Uhde TW, Boulenger JP, Roy-Byrne PP, et al: Longitudinal course of panic disorder: clinical and biological consideration. Prog Neuropsychopharmacol Biol Psychiatry 9:39–51, 1985

van der Kolk BA: The drug treatment of post-traumatic stress disorder. J Affect Disord 13:203–213, 1987

Yehuda R, Giller EL, Southwick SM, et al: Hypothalamic-pituitary-adrenal dysfunction in posttraumatic stress disorder. Biol Psychiatry 30:1031–1048, 1991

Chapter 6

Etiological Factors in the Development of Posttraumatic Stress Disorder

J. Douglas Bremner, M.D.,
Steven M. Southwick, M.D.,
and Dennis S. Charney, M.D.

Society increasingly is forced to grapple with the far-reaching effects of extreme psychological trauma. The unresolved issues of the Vietnam War, for example, have been resurrected in the United States and debates renewed about the meaning of that war for the country. Veterans who continue to be affected by their war experiences are being reexamined in a different light. Concurrently, there has been an increased awareness of severe psychological trauma in the form of criminal victimization and child abuse. Since the inclusion of posttraumatic stress disorder (PTSD) as a diagnosis in DSM-III (American Psychiatric Association 1980), a rapid expansion of research findings has provided objective evidence for the high cost of trauma in terms of psychopathology with associated morbidity and loss of productivity.

Yet, there are a surprising number of unanswered questions about why some people develop PTSD and others do not following exposure to severe psychological trauma. Exposure to a trauma outside the experience of most people is not the only factor involved in the etiology of PTSD. It is clear that there are

We thank Bonnie Green, Ph.D., of Georgetown University School of Medicine and Carolyn M. Mazure, Ph.D., of Yale University School of Medicine for reviewing the manuscript and offering helpful suggestions.

multiple variables that play a role in the development of trauma-related psychopathology. These include antecedents to the stressor, such as genetic constitution, home family life, education, and age. The meaning an event has for an individual, and his or her mental state at the time of the stressor, which may be affected by drug or alcohol intoxication, may also play an important role. Poststressor variables, such as social support, have received increased attention. In addition, it is recognized that the traditional focus on a single stressor neglects the fact that chronic stress also may be an important determinant of PTSD.

Studies in clinical populations support the idea that PTSD is often related to more than a single stressor. For example, in combat veterans, exposure to traumatic stressors is typically repeated many times over the period of combat service. In addition, studies in victims of childhood sexual abuse suggest that these individuals are at increased risk for rape and other forms of sexual assault in later life (Russell 1986; Wyatt et al. 1992). Questions about the role of single versus repeated stressors and the role of nontraumatic factors in the development of PTSD are of crucial importance in understanding the social, cognitive, behavioral, and physiological consequences of exposure to extreme stress. This chapter focuses on epidemiologic and descriptive studies in an effort to delineate specific factors that contribute to the development of PTSD. The reader is referred to previous reviews for information about neurobiological causes of PTSD (Bremner et al. 1993b; Chrousos and Gold 1992). Because most investigations have involved combat veterans, we focus primarily on veteran populations. Recently, however, there has been an increased emphasis on noncombat-related trauma, which we briefly review as it relates to the generalizability of findings related to trauma. In addition, findings from studies at the West Haven Veterans Administration Medical Center (VAMC) on the role of dissociation in the etiology of PTSD are presented and discussed.

SCOPE OF THE PROBLEM

PTSD is a problem of extensive magnitude. More than 20 years after the Vietnam War, 15% of combat veterans continue to suffer from chronic PTSD (Kulka et al. 1990). In addition, nonmilitary violence and stress are increasingly recognized as a major source of morbidity. Data from the Epidemiologic Catchment Area survey suggest that 1% of the general population suffer from PTSD (Helzer et al. 1987). Some authors have noted that this estimate may be artificially low due to the methods of assessment employed (Breslau et al. 1991). For example, using currently accepted methods of assessment, one study of urban young adults found a lifetime PTSD prevalence of 9.2% (Breslau et al. 1991).

WHAT CONSTITUTES A STRESSOR? DEBATE OVER STRESSOR CRITERION

PTSD is unique (with the adjustment disorders) in that included in the diagnostic criteria for the disorder is the requirement that the individual has experienced a significant stressor (Brett et al. 1988). Traditionally, an individual can have all of the symptoms of PTSD, but if an extreme stressor "beyond the range of normal human experience" is not present, then the individual does not meet the full criteria for the disorder.

This traditional stressor criterion for PTSD is problematic for several reasons. Accumulated research suggests that exposure to extreme psychological stress is not uncommon in modern-day society. This raises the question of what constitutes an event as being "beyond the range of normal human experience" (Kilpatrick et al. 1985). Most studies have found a dose-response relationship between the level of stressor intensity and the risk of developing PTSD (for a review, see March 1993). However, the magnitude of the stressor alone does not successfully predict all trauma-related psychopathology (Breslau and Davis 1987a). Discussing the question of the stressor criterion, Breslau and Davis noted that

in DSM-III, the definition of stressors in PTSD implies that in respect to such stressors (and in contrast with other stressors) the potential effects of individual differences on the responsiveness to stressors are obliterated by the overwhelming impact of the stressor. Despite its plausibility, this assumption has little empirical support. (p. 261)

These observations raise questions about the primacy of the stressor in the development of PTSD symptomatology.

Stressors rarely occur in isolation. Emerging evidence reviewed later suggests that individuals with a history of exposure to extreme psychological stress appear to have an increased vulnerability to exposure to subsequent stress. Reconsideration of what some have considered single stressors, such as combat stress, suggests that these events are in fact often episodes of chronic repeated stress that may go on for, in the case of Vietnam War experience, 12 months or more. In addition, there are other factors not directly related to the stressor, such as social support, that may affect the development of PTSD. A consideration of the full range of variables before, during, and after the stressor is necessary to understand why some individuals develop PTSD in response to stress and others do not. What follows is a review of studies related to factors that may affect outcome in individuals exposed to extreme psychological stress.

PRESTRESSOR FACTORS IN
THE DEVELOPMENT OF PTSD

Pretraumatic risk factors for the development of PTSD have long been a subject of interest. Since the time of World War I, the military has attempted to screen recruits for factors that could place individuals at risk for the development of combat-related psychopathology. Predicting who will develop PTSD in response to a stressor has many potential implications for the development of treatment strategies and policy. Findings related to prestressor risk factors have varied widely, in part due to differing methodological approaches.

Premilitary Risk Factors for
Combat-Related PTSD

Freud originally proposed that unresolved psychosexual developmental conflicts predisposed the individual to develop "war neurosis" or what we refer to today as combat-related PTSD. According to Freud, during combat, acute psychiatric symptomatology developed in soldiers who had unresolved conflicts from childhood (Freud et al. 1921). The term *war neurosis* implies that there is an etiology rooted in conflicts related to early development.

The influence of Freud led the military to attempt to predict vulnerability to combat stress based on premilitary developmental variables. Studies of premilitary personality were not able to predict psychopathology following exposure to combat stress (Henderson and Moore 1944). In a study of World War II veterans, 24.5% of acute psychiatric casualties of combat were assessed to have a preexisting diagnosis of neurosis by their own retrospective reporting (Torrie 1944). It is not known, however, how these rates would compare with a carefully matched sample of veterans without a history of combat-related psychopathology. In a study of World War II prisoners of war (POWs), a family history of alcoholism, childhood trauma (including death of parents and chronic physical abuse), and mean age at capture were found to be related to severity of symptoms of war trauma–related PTSD (Speed et al. 1989).

Following the Vietnam War, researchers developed a renewed interest in premilitary risk factors for PTSD. Table 6–1 includes findings related to specific premilitary factors in the development of chronic PTSD following exposure to combat in Vietnam. Younger age at the time of joining the service has been associated with combat-related PTSD; conflicting findings have been noted regarding years of education at the time of joining the service (Table 6–1). Race also has been found in some studies to be predictive of PTSD. Penk et al. (1989) reported increased rates of PTSD in blacks. This increased rate, however, may be accounted for by an increase in exposure to war zone stress in blacks in comparison with whites (B. L. Green et al. 1990a). The National Vietnam Veteran Readjustment Study found increased rates of PTSD in Hispanics. In that study, there was no difference in rates between whites and blacks, after controlling for socioeconomic status (Kulka et al. 1990).

With regard to premilitary personality as a risk factor for PTSD, some studies in Vietnam veterans have shown a relationship between specific variables that are thought to be related to personality, such as low self-esteem in childhood (Card 1987)

Table 6–1. Premilitary risk factors for combat-related posttraumatic stress disorder (PTSD)

Risk factor	Supporting	Refuting
Age at entry	Speed et al. 1989 (II)[a] Worthington 1977 (V)[b] CDC 1988a (V) Hastings 1991 (V) Kulka et al. 1990 (V) True et al. 1988 (V) Fontana and Rosenheck (in press) (V)	Frye and Stockton 1982 (V)
Years of education	Worthington 1977 (V)[b]	Nace et al. 1978 (V)[b,c] Frye and Stockton 1982 (V)
Minority status	Egendorf et al. 1981 (V)[a] CDC 1988a (V) B. L. Green et al. 1990b (V) Kulka et al. 1990 (V) Penk et al. 1989 (V) True et al. 1988 (V)	Card 1983 (V) Helzer et al. 1987 (V)
Socioeconomic status		Nace et al. 1978 (V)[b,c] Frye and Stockton 1982 (V)
Personality problems		Henderson and Moore 1944 (II) Ursano 1981 (V)
Neuroses		Torrie 1944 (II)
Antecedent conflicts		Freud et al. 1921 (I)
Joined the military willingly	Worthington 1978 (V)[b]	
Positive attitude toward the war	Frye and Stockton 1982 (V)	
Premilitary psychiatric illness	Kulka et al. 1990 (V)	Speed et al. 1989 (II)[a]
Emotional stability		Frye and Stockton 1982 (V)

Table 6–1. Premilitary risk factors for combat-related posttraumatic stress disorder (PTSD) *(continued)*

Risk factor	Supporting	Refuting
Social functioning		Foy et al. 1984 (V)
Substance abuse	Kulka et al. 1990 (V) Helzer et al. 1979 (V)[c] Vinokur et al. 1987 (V)	Foy et al. 1984 (V)
Alcohol abuse		Foy and Card 1987 (V) Boman 1986a (V)
Antisocial behavior	Helzer et al. 1987 (V) Kulka et al. 1990 (V) Vinokur et al. 1987 (V)	Resnick et al. 1989 (V) Boman 1986b (V) Bremner et al. 1993b (V)
Legal-authority problems/ criminality		Foy et al. 1984 (V) Nace et al. 1978 (V)[b,c]
Bed-wetting		Boman 1986b (V)
Academic difficulty	Kulka et al. 1990 (V) Helzer et al. 1979 (V)[c] CDC 1988a (V) True et al. 1988 (V) Worthington 1977 (V)[b] Boman 1986b (V) Vinokur et al. 1987 (V)	Card 1983 (V) Foy and Card 1987 (V)
Family psychiatric illness	Davidson et al. 1989 (V) Helzer et al. 1979 (V)[c] Kulka et al. 1990 (V) Vinokur et al. 1987 (V)	Speed et al. 1989 (II)[a]
Family alcoholism	Emery et al. 1991 (V)	Speed et al. 1989 (II)[a] Boman 1986b (V)
Family environment/ stability	Egendorf et al. 1981 (V)[d] Chemtob et al. 1990 (V) Emery et al. 1991 (V) Helzer et al. 1979 (V)[c] Kulka et al. 1990 (V)	Solkoff et al. 1986 (V) Foy et al. 1984 (V) Nace et al. 1978 (V)[b,c] Penk et al. 1981 (V)[b,e] Carroll et al. 1985 (V)
Family employment	Emery et al. 1991 (V)	
Social support		Keane et al. 1985 (V)
Parental support	Vinokur et al. 1987 (V)	

Table 6–1.   Premilitary risk factors for combat-related posttraumatic stress disorder (PTSD) *(continued)*

Risk factor	Supporting	Refuting
Death of parent	Speed et al. 1989 (II)[a]	Bremner et al. 1993a Boman 1986b (V)
Parental separation		Bremner et al. 1993a (V) Boman 1986b (V)
Adoption		Bremner et al. 1993a (V) Boman 1986b (V)
Childhood abuse	Bremner et al. 1993a (V)	Speed et al. 1989 (II)[a] Boman 1986b (V)

Father in combat	Rosenheck and
	  Nathan 1985 (V)
	Fontana and Rosenheck
	  (in press) (V)	

Previous combat stress reaction	Solomon et al. 1987a (Isr) Solomon et al. 1987b (Isr)	

Note.   II = World War II studies; V = Vietnam War studies; I = World War I studies; CDC = Centers for Disease Control; Isr = Israeli wars studies.
[a]Subjects were prisoners of war.
[b]Used measures of general function as an outcome measure.
[c]Used depression as an outcome measure.
[d]Used non-DSM-III or DSM-III-R criteria for PTSD as an outcome measure.
[e]Subjects were PTSD patients seeking treatment for substance abuse.

and external locus of control (Frye and Stockton 1982; Vinokur et al. 1987), and the subsequent development of PTSD. In other studies, however, premilitary adjustment has not been associated with the development of combat-related PTSD (Foy and Card 1987; Ursano 1981). Studies of premilitary antisocial behavior as a risk factor have been conflicting, with some studies suggesting that a history of antisocial behavior in childhood increases the risk for combat-related PTSD (Helzer et al. 1987; Kulka et al. 1990); another study found no association between childhood antisocial behavior and PTSD (Resnick et al. 1989). In addition to PTSD, depression following combat exposure in Vietnam has been associated with premilitary antisocial behavior, alcoholism, parental arrest, narcotic use, and failure to graduate from high school (Helzer et al. 1976, 1979). Other factors that have been associated with the development of combat-related PTSD include premilitary Minnesota Multiphasic Personality Inventory score (Schnurr et al. 1993) and premilitary psychiatric illness (Kulka et al. 1990).

Conflicting results have also been obtained relating to the role of family environment in the development of combat-related PTSD. General measures of family environment (Egendorf et al. 1981), as well as factors such as family alcoholism (Davidson et al. 1985; Emery et al. 1991) and parental unemployment (Emery et al. 1991), have been associated with an increased risk for developing combat-related PTSD. Poor family relationships and a lack of family closeness have also been shown to increase risk (Chemtob et al. 1990). Premilitary social support has not been associated with combat-related PTSD (Keane et al. 1985). Family environment measured by general indexes has been shown to be predictive of PTSD by some authors but not others; several studies have found a relationship between academic performance and PTSD (see Table 6–1). One group combined parental supportiveness, parental problems such as psychiatric illness, alcoholism and substance abuse, and serving time in jail with subjective behavior problems such as academic difficulties, trouble with the law, alcohol and substance abuse, and antisocial activity and found them to be predictive of combat-related PTSD (Vinokur et al. 1987). Having a father who was in combat has been associated with increased risk for PTSD (Rosenheck 1986; Rosenheck and Nathan 1985), possibly secondary to the fact that these individuals may have entered the military at a younger age and participated in atrocities during the war (Fontana and Rosenheck, in press).

Recently, the role of previous exposure to stress in the development of PTSD after subsequent exposure to an extreme stressor has received increased attention. We have compared rates of childhood physical abuse and other stressful or potentially predisposing variables in Vietnam combat veterans with PTSD with those in Vietnam combat veterans without PTSD. A significantly greater number of PTSD patients had a history of childhood physical abuse (26%) than non-PTSD combat veterans

(7%). In addition, there was no relationship between other stressful and potentially predisposing events and PTSD in that study (Bremner et al. 1993a), suggesting that a history of exposure to physical abuse in childhood increases the risk for combat-related PTSD. In summary, many studies to date suggest that a stressful, chaotic environment in childhood, which is associated with poor family support and closeness, antisocial behavior, poor academic performance, mental illness, and alcohol and substance abuse in the veteran, predisposes the individual to the development of combat-related PTSD. Mental illness, alcohol and substance abuse, and economic instability in the family also have been shown to increase the risk for the development of combat-related PTSD. Many other studies, however, do not support a relationship between premilitary factors and combat-related PTSD. Prospective longitudinal study designs that attempt to utilize these factors in the prediction of PTSD could help answer these questions.

Repeated Exposure to Combat Stress in the Israeli wars and Desert Storm

Studies from veterans of other wars suggest that individuals may vary in their susceptibility to combat stress. Soldiers of the Israeli wars with a history of acute combat stress reactions during previous wars were found to be at an increased risk for development of combat stress in response to subsequent conflicts in comparison with soldiers without a history of combat stress reaction in previous wars. In fact, soldiers with a prior history of combat stress reaction were more likely to experience combat stress reaction in the current conflict than recruits with no prior history of combat exposure (Solomon et al. 1987a, 1987b). Female veterans of Desert Storm with high levels of symptomatology related to previous Vietnam combat exposure also have been shown to have higher levels of distress after Desert Storm than female Desert Storm veterans with low levels of symptomatology related to previous Vietnam combat exposure (Wolfe et al. 1992). These studies suggest that a history of prior stress reaction is associated with an increased vulnerability on exposure to subsequent stress.

Prestressor Risk Factors for PTSD
Related to Civilian Trauma

Evidence from individuals exposed to civilian trauma is consistent with a role for prestressor variables in the development of psychopathology following exposure to trauma. Women presenting to a rape clinic have been shown to have a higher rate of previous exposure to rape than matched control subjects (reviewed in Finkelhor et al. 1986). In a study of urban young adults, the authors found a 39.1% lifetime prevalence of exposure to traumatic events, with risk factors for exposure including low education, male sex, early conduct problems, extraversion, and a family history of psychiatric disorder or substance abuse (Breslau and Davis 1992; Breslau et al. 1991). The rate of PTSD in those exposed to a traumatic stressor was 23.6%. Factors that increased the risk of PTSD following exposure were an early history of parental separation (3.5 times increased risk) and preexisting anxiety or depression (2.5 times increased risk) (Breslau et al. 1991). In a study of firefighters exposed to a bushfire disaster, risk for development of chronic PTSD was increased by a history of premorbid adverse life events and premorbid psychiatric disorder. Neuroticism and a tendency to avoid thinking through aversive experiences also predicted the development of chronic PTSD (McFarlane et al. 1988a, 1988b). These studies suggest that specific factors, such as a previous history of stress and previous psychiatric disorders, may increase the risk of exposure to a traumatic stressor as well as the development of PTSD.

Hypotheses Related to the Role of Premorbid
Factors for the Development of PTSD

There are several hypotheses related to the role of premorbid factors in the development of PTSD. These are perhaps best categorized under the headings of stress evaporation versus residual stress and stress inoculation versus stress sensitization.

Stress evaporation versus residual stress. The stress evaporation theory holds that preservice and/or postservice variables are of primary importance in determining the symptoms with which the combat veteran presents during the first several years after combat exposure. Any symptoms that are secondary to the combat itself evaporate within a relatively short period of time (Worthington 1978). The second theory, the residual stress theory, gives primary importance to the stress of combat itself and claims that combat stress does have a significant effect on the individual at the current time (Figley 1978). The results of several large epidemiologic studies conducted during the 1980s on veterans of the Vietnam War are consistent with this theory (Centers for Disease Control 1988a, 1988b; Egendorf et al. 1981; Kulka et al. 1990). However, there is renewed interest in the question of what determines why some individuals develop PTSD, whereas others with an equivalent level of exposure to combat stress do not.

Stress inoculation versus stress sensitization. There are two conflicting theories regarding the effects of prior stress exposure on the response to current stress. One theory, sometimes referred to as the stress inoculation theory, suggests that a history of prior exposure to stress strengthens the individual's coping and promotes resilience in the face of adversity (Coleman et al. 1980). The other theory, sometimes referred to as the stress sensitization theory, suggests that repeated stress results in depleted resources, making the individual more susceptible when confronted with later stress (Selye 1956; Silver et al. 1980). Results from Vietnam combat veterans with a history of childhood abuse and Israeli veterans of more than one war are consistent with the theory that repeated exposure to stress has a cumulative negative effect; soldiers with a prior history of negative effects to stress are at increased risk to have a negative response to future stress. Another possible interpretation of the findings of reactivation of stress disorders from the Israeli wars is that certain individuals are genetically vulnerable to the effects of stress. This explanation places the causative role in the inherent constitution of the subject rather than in the effects of previous stressors.

Role of genetic and familial factors. One area that has been the subject of recent investigation is genetic susceptibility to the effects of extreme stress. In a study of urban young adults, individuals with a family history of anxiety were 2.9 times more likely to develop PTSD than other individuals who also had been exposed to a traumatic stressor. A family history of antisocial behavior also increased the risk of PTSD by 2.1 times, and a family history of depression was not associated with PTSD (Breslau et al. 1991). In a study of monozygotic twins with and without a history of Vietnam combat service, twins with a history of heavy combat in Vietnam were 9 times more likely currently to be diagnosed with PTSD than their noncombat twin (Goldberg et al. 1990). Increased rates of alcoholism and anxiety have been found in family members of Vietnam veterans with PTSD in comparison with control subjects (Davidson et al. 1985). In a small sample of Vietnam veterans, rates of psychiatric disorders were increased in the children of patients with PTSD in comparison with control subjects, with the most common disorder being attention deficit disorder (Davidson et al. 1989). Considering the symptom overlap between PTSD and attention deficit disorder of hyperarousal and decreased concentration, these findings are potentially of interest. In summary, studies related to genetic and familial contributions to PTSD are still in their infancy, and although some interesting evidence has been accumulated, it is too early at this time to draw conclusions in this area.

PERITRAUMATIC FACTORS IN THE DEVELOPMENT OF PTSD

Accumulated research suggests that the traumatic stressor has primary importance in the development of PTSD. Evidence supports a relationship between trauma and PTSD, with a remarkable conservation of symptomatology across stressor type, population, and age at the time of exposure (Eaton et al. 1982; Finkelhor et al. 1986; Foy et al. 1984; Herman et al. 1986; Gleser et al. 1981; Kulka et al. 1990; Pynoos et al. 1987).

Military Risk Factors for Development of Combat-Related PTSD

The role of combat stressors in the development of PTSD. The importance of combat-related stressors in the development of what is known today as combat-related PTSD has been recognized since the time of World War I (Table 6–2). In a study of British soldiers in the North African campaign of World War II, exposure to overwhelming combat stressors, such as incoming mortar fire or the witnessing of a close friend being killed, in addition to factors such as "heat, sun, and flies," was described as a precipitant of acute psychiatric disorder. The important effects of morale and social support within the unit on the development of combat-related psychopathology were also noted (Torrie 1944). Other reports from World War II have established a relationship between exposure to combat stress and long-term psychiatric symptomatology currently categorized as part of PTSD (Henderson and Moore 1944) as well as other symptoms, including depression and momentary blackouts (Archibald and Tuddenham 1965). Follow-up investigations of World War II and Korean POWs have found increased rates of death from suicide (Nefzger 1970) and increased levels of psychopathology in POWs in comparison with control subjects (Beebe 1975). A study of World War II POWs indicated several factors related to captivity to be significantly associated with the outcome of PTSD, including losing weight, having nightmares during internment, being forced to relocate, being a witness to torture, experiencing mental suffering, and being injured while in captivity (Speed et al. 1989).

With Vietnam War veterans, a relationship has been established between the level of exposure to combat stress and degree of PTSD symptomatology by several investigators (Borus 1973; Centers for Disease Control 1988a, 1988b; Escobar et al. 1983; B. L. Green et al. 1989; Kulka et al. 1990; Laufer et al. 1985a, 1985b; True et al. 1988; see also Boyle et al. 1989; Foy et al. 1987). A positive relationship between degree of traumatic stressor during imprisonment and development of psychiatric disorders has been found in a group of U.S. Air Force POWs from the Vietnam War (Ursano et al. 1981). Also, studies of veterans of Desert Storm are consistent with a relationship between severity of combat trauma and long-term psychopathology (Southwick et al. 1993).

The relationship between particular traumatic events and individual responses to trauma has also been addressed. Specific elements of combat-related stressors have been found to be of importance in the determination of outcome, including being

Table 6–2. Peritraumatic risk factors for combat-related posttraumatic stress disorder

Risk factor	Supporting	Refuting
Combat exposure[a]	Archibald et al. 1962 (II) Breslau and Davis 1987b (V) Card 1983 (V) Egendorf et al. 1981 (V) Foy et al. 1984 (V) Gallers et al. 1988 (V) B. L. Green et al. 1990a (V) Kulka et al. 1990 (V) Laufer et al. 1985a, 1985b (V) True et al. 1988 (V)	
Injured in combat/captivity	Solkoff et al. 1986 (V) Speed et al. 1989 (II)[b] Card 1983 (V)	Frye and Stockton 1982 (V) Breslau and Davis 1987b (V)
Observing deaths of others	Solkoff et al. 1986 (V) Card 1983 (V)	
Killing others	Solkoff et al. 1986 (V) Card 1983 (V)	
Friends killed	Solkoff et al. 1986 (V) Breslau and Davis 1987b (V) Chemtob et al. 1990 (V)	
Guilt over the death of a friend	Chemtob et al. 1990 (V)	
Surrounded by the enemy		Breslau and Davis 1987b (V)
Unit patrol	B. L. Green et al. 1989 (V)	
Months in combat	Solkoff et al. 1986 (V)	Card 1983 (V)
Threat to life	Card 1983 (V)	Frye and Stockton 1982 (V)
Attached to a South Vietnamese unit	Breslau and Davis 1987b (V)	

Table 6–2.   Peritraumatic risk factors for combat-related posttraumatic stress disorder *(continued)*

Risk factor	Supporting	Refuting
Participation in/ witnessing of atrocities	Laufer et al. 1985a, 1985b (V)[c] T. Yager et al. 1984 (V) Breslau and Davis 1987b (V) B. L. Green et al. 1990a (V) Kulka et al. 1990 (V) Yehuda et al. 1992 (V) Fontana and Rosenheck (in press) (V) Speed et al. 1989 (II)[b] B. L. Green et al. 1989 (V)	
Receiving a disciplinary action	Foy et al. 1984 (V) Worthington 1977 (V)[d] Gallers et al. 1988 (V)	Card 1983 (V)
Dissociation during trauma	Spiegel et al. 1988 (V) Cardeña and Spiegel 1993 (V) Bremner et al. 1992 (V) Fontana and Rosenheck (in press) (V)	
Alcohol abuse	Card 1983 (V)	Boman 1986a (V)
Substance abuse	Gallers et al. 1988 (V)	Card 1983 (V)
Military adjustment	Foy et al. 1984 (V)	
Emotional preparedness to leave unit	Chemtob et al. 1990 (V)	
External locus of control	Frye and Stockton 1982 (V) Vinokur et al. 1987 (V)	

Note.   V = Vietnam War studies; II = World War II studies.
[a]Listed are some of the many studies reporting a relationship between combat exposure and PTSD.
[b]Subjects were prisoners of war.
[c]Used non-DSM-III or DSM-III-R criteria for PTSD as an outcome measure.
[d]Used measures of general function as an outcome measure.

injured in combat, observing the deaths of others, having friends killed, being involved in killing others, and serving greater length of time in combat (Solkoff et al. 1986).

The role of atrocities in the development of PTSD. Some authors have noted an important role for participation in or witnessing of atrocities in the development of psychopathology in Vietnam veterans (Breslau and Davis 1987b; Fontana and Rosenheck, in press; B. L. Green et al. 1990b; Kulka et al. 1990; Laufer et al. 1985a, 1985b; T. Yager et al. 1984; Yehuda et al. 1992). Participation in atrocities has also been associated with increased marijuana and heroin use as well as self-reported stress (T. Yager et al. 1984). A sample of 69 psychiatric inpatients showed that having a buddy killed, participating in and witnessing atrocities, and being separated from one's unit were all associated with an increased risk for PTSD. After differences in level of combat exposure were controlled, participation in atrocities was still associated with an increased risk for the development of PTSD (Breslau and Davis et al. 1987b). In addition, the type of atrocity to which the individual was exposed has been found to affect outcome differentially. Participation in atrocities was most commonly associated with cognitive disruption (including difficulties thinking and difficulties with memory); witnessing of atrocities and combat exposure were associated with intrusive symptomatology (Laufer et al. 1985a, 1985b).

Dissociation and etiology of PTSD: findings from research at the West Haven VAMC. The past few years have seen an increased interest in the role of dissociation in the development of PTSD, partially related to a rediscovery of the theoretical contributions of Pierre Janet (Nemiah 1989; van der Kolk and van der Hart 1989). This interest has been accompanied by a rapid expansion of research in the area of dissociation and trauma. Further, several studies of hypnotizability (Spiegel et al. 1988; Stutman and Bliss 1985) and dissociative symptomatology (Branscomb 1991; Loewenstein and Putnam 1988) have found evidence that supports a relationship between dissociation and PTSD.

In a series of studies at the West Haven VAMC, we have examined the relationship between dissociation and trauma in

Vietnam combat veterans with and without PTSD (Table 6–3). In our initial study, 53 Vietnam combat veterans with PTSD were found to have increased levels of general dissociative symptomatology as measured by the Dissociative Experiences Scale (DES; Bernstein and Putnam 1986) in comparison with 32 Vietnam combat veterans without PTSD. Mean ± SD DES score in that study was 27 ± 18 for PTSD patients in comparison with 13.7 ± 16 for the non-PTSD subjects. The difference in DES score between the two groups persisted after controlling for level of combat exposure using analysis of covariance (Bremner et al. 1992). This study showed that an increase in dissociative symptomatology is

Table 6–3. The role of dissociation in the etiology of posttraumatic stress disorder (PTSD): findings from the West Haven Veterans Administration Medical Center

Finding	Instrument(s)	Reference(s)
Increased dissociative symptomatology	DES, SCID-D, CADSS	Bremner et al. 1992, 1993b; J. D. Bremner, unpublished data, June 1994
Increased dissociative symptoms with combat and postmilitary trauma	DEQ-M	Bremner et al. 1992; J. D. Bremner, unpublished data, June 1994
Dissociation during combat trauma associated with long-term course of PTSD symptoms and associated psychopathology	DEQ-M, Mississippi, DES, BSI	Bremner et al. 1992; J. D. Bremner unpublished data, June 1994
Increased dissociative states with traumatic reminders	CADSS	J. D. Bremner, unpublished data, June 1994

Note. DES = Dissociative Experiences Scale; SCID-D = Structured Clinical Interview for DSM-III-R–Dissociative Disorders; CADSS = Clinician Administered Dissociative States Scale; DEQ-M = Dissociative Experiences Questionnaire; Mississippi = Mississippi Scale for Combat-Related PTSD; BSI = Brief Symptom Inventory.

associated with PTSD and is not a nonspecific outcome associated with exposure to combat trauma alone.

In a second study, 40 Vietnam combat veterans with PTSD were compared with 15 Vietnam combat veterans without PTSD for dissociative symptomatology in specific symptom areas using the Structured Clinical Interview for DSM-III-R—Dissociative Disorders (Steinberg et al. 1990). PTSD patients had higher levels of dissociation in each of the five symptom areas measured by this instrument: amnesia, depersonalization, derealization, identity confusion, and identity alteration (Bremner et al. 1993c).

We have also been interested in the relationship between dissociative symptomatology at the time of traumatic events and long-term psychopathology. Vietnam combat veterans with and without PTSD were asked to describe their most traumatic premilitary, combat-related, and postmilitary traumatic event, and the dissociative states associated with those events were evaluated retrospectively using a modification of the Dissociative Experiences Questionnaire (C. Marmar, unpublished questionnaire). Of PTSD patients, 41% reported death of a friend as their most traumatic combat-related event, compared with 15% of non-PTSD veterans ($P < .05$). Of non-PTSD veterans, 30% reported an extreme threat to their safety as their most traumatic combat-related event, in comparison with 3% of PTSD patients ($P < .05$).

There were no differences between groups in frequency of reporting for other combat-related traumas (J. D. Bremner, unpublished observations, June 1994). Vietnam combat veterans with PTSD had an increase in dissociative states at the time of combat-related (Bremner et al. 1992) and postmilitary traumatic events (J. D. Bremner, unpublished observations, June 1994) in comparison with Vietnam combat veterans without PTSD. There were no differences in dissociative states at the time of premilitary traumatic events between the two groups (J. D. Bremner, unpublished observations, June 1994). Dissociation at the time of combat trauma as measured by the Dissociative Experiences Questionnaire was found to be strongly associated with outcome in terms of long-term PTSD symptomatology as measured by the Mississippi Scale for Combat-Related PTSD (Keane et al. 1988) after controlling for other factors, including level of combat exposure, participation in atrocities, and months in Vietnam (Bremner et al. 1992). There was a significant correlation between dissociation during combat-related trauma and long-term psychopathology as measured by the Brief Symptom Inventory, PTSD symptomatology as measured by the Mississippi Scale, and general dissociative symptomatology as measured by the DES. In addition, there was a significant association between dissociation during combat-related trauma and dissociation during subsequent postmilitary traumatic events (J. D. Bremner, unpublished observations, June 1994).

In an independent follow-up study, we developed an instrument for the measurement of dissociative states at specific time points: the Clinician Administered Dissociative States Scale (CADSS). We found significantly increased levels of dissociative states at baseline as measured by the CADSS in Vietnam combat veterans with PTSD compared with Vietnam combat veterans without PTSD, psychiatric patients with schizophrenia and affective disorders, and healthy control subjects. PTSD patients also had a significant increase in dissociative symptoms from baseline as measured by the CADSS following exposure to traumatic reminders (J. D. Bremner, unpublished observations, June 1994)

These findings suggest that dissociative responses to trauma may play a role in PTSD. Previously, some clinicians (Spiegel and Cardeña 1991) have speculated that dissociation may be a defense mechanism that protects the individual from potentially harmful aspects of psychological trauma. Our findings suggest that dissociative responses to trauma are actually associated with a worse outcome as measured by long-term PTSD, general psychiatric, and dissociative symptomatology. Further, dissociative responses to trauma may play a role in the development of PTSD. Alternatively, dissociative responses to trauma may be a marker of poor outcome or a characteristic of individuals who are at high risk for the development of long-term PTSD and general psychiatric symptomatology.

Peristressor Factors Related to Development of PTSD Following Exposure to Civilian Trauma

Studies in victims of nonmilitary trauma also support a relationship between degree of traumatization and severity of long-term psychopathology. Female victims of rape, robbery, and assault have been found to have increased levels of psychopathology in comparison with females who have not been victimized (Kilpatrick et al. 1985). Increased rates of PTSD, as high as 35%, have been found in samples of women exposed to rape and related crimes compared with control subjects (Resnick et al. 1992). Individuals exposed to violent crimes, deaths, or accidents have a current rate of PTSD of 7%–11%. In comparison with other events, sexual assault is associated with the highest rate of PTSD (Norris 1992). In addition, studies of exposure to natural disasters (Gleser et al. 1981; B. L. Green et al. 1992), fire (B. L. Green et al. 1985), and childhood abuse (Carmen et al. 1984; Swett et al. 1990; reviewed in Finkelhor et al. 1986) support a relationship between the severity of traumatic exposure and long-term psychopathology. Increased levels of dissociative symptomatology have been associated with exposure to the civilian trauma of an earthquake (Cardeña and Spiegel 1993) and childhood abuse (Chu and Dill 1990) and have been associated with populations, such as Cambodian refugees, with a history of high levels of traumatization (Carlson and Rosser-Hogan 1991). Studies of victims of the Buffalo Creek Dam flood in Buffalo Creek Valley, West Virginia, which occurred February 1972, show a lifetime prevalence of PTSD of 59.4%, with the next most common diagnosis being major depression (35.8%), followed by generalized anxiety disorder (17.6%), and simple phobia (15.6%) (B. L. Green et al. 1992).

Hypotheses Related to Role of Peritraumatic Factors for the Development of PTSD

Importance of life threat.   Extreme threat to life has been hypothesized to be a key factor in the long-term consequences of stress (Chrousos and Gold 1992). Life threat and physical injury appear to play an important role in determining the risk for the development of PTSD (March 1993). Experimental studies of the effects of stress use paradigms in which animals are exposed to life-threatening situations. These include cats being exposed to dogs, and rats being exposed to electric shock, suspended in water, immobilized, or exposed to extreme cold, as well as other situations that are perceived by the animal as life threatening. Exposure to life threat in animals results in a variety of behavioral and neurobiological effects that parallel the effects of stress on humans (Bremner et al. 1993b). These findings suggest that life threat may represent a key factor in the development of psychopathology following exposure to extreme stress.

Studies in civilian trauma also support a role for threat to life in the development of psychopathology following extreme stress. In female victims of crime such as rape, subjective perception of threat to life appears to be associated with long-term psychopathology. This may explain why many women who experience noncompleted crimes, in which the perception of a possible threat to life is higher, have worse outcome in comparison with women who experience completed crimes. For instance, women who have been the victim of a successful robbery appear to be less disturbed in relation to the event than women for whom the robbery was interrupted for some reason; this is apparently because of the quality of the unknown related to an uncompleted robbery (Kilpatrick et al. 1985). Life threat may represent the common feature that explains similar outcomes to different types of stressors.

Influence of alcohol and substance abuse.   Another area of interest to researchers is the relationship between alcohol and substance abuse and the development of PTSD. An increase in both alcohol and substance abuse has been associated with the diagnosis of PTSD in both veteran populations (Atkinson et al. 1982; Boman 1986a, 1986b; Escobar et al. 1983; Faustman and White 1989; Kulka et al. 1990; Sierles et al. 1983; True et al. 1988) and civilian populations (Helzer et al. 1987). Some authors have found premilitary substance abuse (Helzer et al. 1979; Kulka et al. 1990; Vinokur et al. 1987), but not alcohol abuse (Foy and Card 1987), to be a risk factor for the development of combat-related PTSD. It is possible that an association between alcohol and substance abuse and PTSD could be explained by the fact that intoxication during exposure to trauma increases the risk of developing trauma-related psychopathology. Another explanation is that alcohol and substance abuse follow the development of PTSD, possibly because of a tendency on the part of patients with

PTSD to self-medicate. Consistent with this idea, exposure to extremely stressful combat-related events in the form of atrocities has been found to be associated with an increased use of heroin and marijuana among Vietnam combat veterans (T. Yager et al. 1984).

It is also possible that there is no relationship between PTSD and alcohol and substance abuse. Increased rates of alcohol and substance abuse are associated with all mental disorders, especially in treatment-seeking populations, and it is not clear that these rates are increased in PTSD relevant to other disorders. Consistent with this, one study found no increase in alcohol dependence in all veterans in comparison with the general population after controlling for socioeconomic factors (Boscarino 1981). Finally, research has not found a direct association between combat exposure and drug and alcohol abuse in Vietnam combat veterans seeking treatment for their disorders (Fontana and Rosenheck, in press). Further research is indicated to clarify the relationship between drug and alcohol abuse and PTSD.

Individual meaning and horror of war.   Early theoreticians postulated that the meaning of the stressful event was more important than the objectively defined magnitude of the event (Freud et al. 1921). The role of meaning in the response to stress continues to be a subject of interest up to the present day (Lazarus 1984; J. Yager 1975). Multiple factors, which are naturally difficult to quantify, determine what a particular event means for the individual. For example, for someone who had lost a brother from an accidental fire in childhood, seeing a friend become burned during combat may be particularly upsetting and may renew unresolved feelings related to the original accidental death. Unresolved issues of aggression in childhood may be brought into full relief during combat when aggression is both expected and often rewarded.

POSTSTRESSOR FACTORS IN THE DEVELOPMENT OF PTSD

One of the unique aspects of the Vietnam War was the intense controversy about the goals of the war and the justification for the involvement of the United States in the conflict. Veterans returning from the Vietnam War received little or no support on returning home, often being ridiculed. There were virtually none of the ticker-tape parades that greeted veterans of World War I and World War II. In addition, it is now recognized that many victims of nonmilitary traumas, such as rape, have been exposed to various forms of secondary traumatization or upsetting events that occur after the trauma and exacerbate the effects of the original trauma. Inadequate social support is increasingly recognized as an important modifier of the long-term effects of trauma.

Postmilitary Risk Factors for Combat-Related PTSD

Some authors have suggested that a lack of social support may play a role in the development of combat-related PTSD in veterans returning from the war. A survey of 1,089 Veterans Administration mental health professionals soon after the withdrawal of American forces from Vietnam found that most treaters felt that Vietnam veterans were not as well adjusted as veterans of previous wars. In addition, treaters with the most contact with PTSD patients were more likely to state that the social support system on the veterans' return home was critically important in the development of the stress disorder (Keane and Fairbank 1983).

Other groups have found that Vietnam veterans with PTSD were more likely to perceive that they received little social support from friends and family on returning home and experienced more changes in their environment on returning home than those without PTSD (Solkoff et al. 1986). One study found that Vietnam veterans with the support of a spouse had lower levels of symptomatology than unmarried veterans (Card 1983). The National Vietnam Veteran Readjustment Study found an association between level of social support after the war and the development of PTSD (Kulka et al. 1990). In a sample of Hispanic Vietnam veterans, level of PTSD symptomatology was correlated with acculturation and social network, although this study does not answer questions about cause and effect (Escobar et al. 1983). Frye and Stockton (1982) found that the veterans' perception of family helpfulness on returning home accounted for a greater percentage of the variance in a model for the prediction of PTSD than all other factors, including level of combat exposure. In summary, there are now several studies that consistently support a role for lack of social support in the development of combat-related PTSD (Table 6–4).

One question these studies raise is the degree to which social support after the war was of primary importance in the development of PTSD. It is possible that low social support is related to other factors, such as being raised in a home where childhood abuse and neglect is prevalent, and that these events rather than social support per se resulted in a predisposition to the development of PTSD. An important question is whether individuals exposed to an extreme stress are more likely to become exposed to subsequent stressors. Put another way, do patients with combat-related PTSD have an increase in stressful and traumatic

Table 6–4.   Postmilitary risk factors for combat-related posttraumatic stress disorder (PTSD)

Risk factor	Supporting	Refuting
Social support	Keane and Fairbank 1983 Solkoff et al. 1986 Escobar et al. 1983 Kulka et al. 1990 Frye and Stockton 1982 Vinokur et al. 1987	
Socioeconomic status		Frye and Stockton 1982
Marital status	Card 1983	
Alcohol abuse	Foy and Card 1987 Kulka et al. 1990	
Substance abuse	Card 1983 Foy and Card 1987 Kulka et al. 1990	
Immediacy of discharge from the military	Frye and Stockton 1982	

Note. All studies were on Vietnam veterans.

events throughout life (Speed et al. 1989)?

Some authors have shown an increase in stressful life events in PTSD patients after the war. A relationship between stressful life events, particularly personal loss, and depressive disorders has been found (Cadoret et al. 1972; Ghaziuddin et al. 1990; Paykel et al. 1975; Warheit 1979). One study of Vietnam combat veterans found a significant correlation between current number and severity of stressful life events and current diagnosis of PTSD (M. A. Green and Berlin 1987). A relationship between high levels of combat and exposure to atrocities during combat and negative life events after the war has also been shown (B. L. Green et al. 1990b). In our sample of 61 Vietnam War combat veterans with PTSD, there was no relationship between the number of stressful life events based on the format of Paykel et al. (1975) and the level of PTSD symptomatology in any of the 2-year intervals after Vietnam (Bremner et al., in press). It is possible, however, that these patients had high levels of symptomatology that were not easily affected by subsequent stressful life events. Patients with PTSD appear to have high levels of stress and trauma throughout life. It is likely that future studies will show a relationship between PTSD and total lifetime stressful and traumatic events.

Poststressor Factors Related to Development of PTSD Following Civilian Trauma

The response to victims of civilian trauma such as rape could modify long-term outcome following the trauma. Rape victims in many instances have been subjected to a demeaning and stigmatizing review by a male-dominated judicial system. Some victims have been told that rape victims encourage their assailants by "provocative" behavior. Most victims feel shame and guilt, which discourage them from talking openly about their feelings and seeking support. These factors all contribute to a decrease in potential social support for victims of civilian trauma, such as rape, in a manner analogous to that of combat veterans with PTSD. Future studies are indicated to examine the relationship between poststressor variables such as social support and outcome following exposure to civilian traumas.

Hypotheses Related to Role of Posttraumatic Factors for Development of PTSD

Combat veterans with high levels of combat exposure tend to seek out their fellow veterans to a greater degree than veterans with low levels of combat exposure (Elder and Clipp 1988). It appears that veterans of previous wars have naturally aggregated toward a medium that is beneficial in helping them to cope with trauma: meeting others who shared common experiences, talking about traumatic events, and having a forum for their grief. It is possible that individuals who do not have such an opportunity may not do as well following exposure to trauma. Incidents incurred by the negative reactions that veterans of the Vietnam War received on returning home, such as being denied membership in veterans organizations such as the Veterans of Foreign Wars, may have deprived veterans of the chance to ventilate their feelings in a supportive and understanding environment.

Talking about trauma has been shown to affect outcome following exposure to trauma. It is significant, therefore, that Vietnam veterans with PTSD have been found to have significantly more problems with self-disclosure and assertiveness than veterans without PTSD, although they show no differences on other measures of affection and intimacy (Carroll et al. 1985). Shame, guilt, the feeling of not being understood, and other factors all contribute to hinder the process of talking about feelings and thoughts related to trauma and seeking support, which is so important in modifying the negative consequences of exposure to trauma.

CONCLUSION

It is easy to be lulled into a false perception that because the "cause" of the disorder is included within DSM-IV (American Psychiatric Association 1994) diagnostic criteria for PTSD, there are no questions remaining to be answered about the etiology of PTSD. In fact, it has been shown that there are numerous factors that affect the development of PTSD in response to trauma. Several studies have shown that social support after exposure to a stressor affects outcome. Individuals who do not perceive that they are supported by family, friends, and the community at large have been found to have more PTSD symptomatology than individuals who have adequate social support. Young age at the time of joining the military, minority status, antisocial behavior in childhood, and premilitary psychiatric status have been shown to be associated with the development of combat-related PTSD by some investigators, whereas no association has been shown by others. A few studies have shown that exposure to premilitary stressors, such as childhood physical abuse, may increase the risk for the development of PTSD following exposure to a traumatic stressor. Factors that are related to abuse and neglect, such as family alcoholism and mental illness, poverty, antisocial behavior, and poor academic performance, have also been associated with the development of combat-related PTSD. These findings, however, are from small samples and require replication.

Preliminary investigations are starting to use approaches such as path analyses to examine how variables that occur before, during, and after the stressor combine to determine the final outcome (Fontana and Rosenheck, in press). For instance, age at the time of joining the military and years of education have been found to predict combat exposure, and high levels of combat exposure have been associated with PTSD (B. L. Green et al. 1990b). One study combined several premilitary, military, and postmilitary factors into one model to predict outcome correctly in 90% of cases. These factors included a negative perception of family helpfulness on return home, high level of combat exposure, external locus of control, immediate discharge after the war, and a positive attitude toward the Vietnam War before entering the military (Frye and Stockton 1982). Methods that examine multiple prestressor, peristressor, and poststressor variables will clearly be useful in future research.

A cumulative lifetime history of trauma may be an important determinant of the development of PTSD. At one time, prior trauma was considered by some to increase the resilience of the individual to subsequent traumas. This hypothesis, the stress inoculation theory, held that previous exposure to stress reduced the risk of pathology with subsequent reexposure. Emerging research evidence is not consistent with an increase in resiliency resulting from exposure to physical abuse in childhood. Rather, the data support the stress sensitization theory, which holds that exposure to repeated stress makes the individual more susceptible to the effects of stress. Research also suggests that veterans with combat-related PTSD may have been exposed to an increase in stressful events since the war. Future studies may find that PTSD is related to an increase in stressful events throughout life and not just to the defined criterion A stressor. Captured by the popular notion of the "walking disaster" or "the disaster waiting to happen," some individuals seem to be at an increased risk for exposure to trauma. This could be a result of a chaotic and dysfunctional family history, limited socioeconomic opportunity, the lifestyle of a substance-abusing person, or behavior patterns that are a consequence of exposure to stress that make the individual more vulnerable to exposure to future stress. We have observed, for instance, that many Vietnam combat veterans with PTSD frequently go into dangerous neighborhoods with little regard for their own safety. Future studies are indicated to examine the hypothesis that an increase in lifetime trauma is associated with particular individuals.

Understanding the factors that influence the development of PTSD in response to a stressor may be useful in the treatment and prevention of PTSD. Considering the magnitude of the problem, information about what determines who gets PTSD following exposure to trauma could play an important role in reducing the negative long-term consequences of extreme stress.

REFERENCES

American Psychiatric Association: Diagnostic and Statistical Manual, 3rd Edition. Washington, DC, American Psychiatric Association, 1980

American Psychiatric Association: Diagnostic and Statistical Manual, 4th Edition. Washington, DC, American Psychiatric Association, 1994

Archibald HC, Tuddenham RD: Persistent stress reaction after combat. Arch Gen Psychiatry 12:475–481, 1965

Atkinson RM, Henderson RG, Sparr LF, et al: Assessment of Vietnam veterans for posttraumatic stress disorder in veterans administration disability claims. Am J Psychiatry 139:118–121, 1982

Beebe GW: Follow-up studies of World War II and Korean war prisoners. Am J Epidemiol 101:400–422, 1975

Bernstein E, Putnam T: Development, reliability, and validity of a dissociation scale. J Nerv Ment Dis 174:727–735, 1986

Boman B: Combat stress, posttraumatic stress disorder, and associated psychiatric disturbance. Psychosomatics 27:567–573, 1986a

Boman B: Early experiential environment, maternal bonding, and the susceptibility to posttraumatic stress disorder. Mil Med 151:528–530, 1986b

Borus JF: Reentry; I: adjustment issues facing the Vietnam returnee. Arch Gen Psychiatry 28:501–506, 1973

Boscarino J: Patterns of alcohol use among veterans and nonveterans: a confirmation of previous findings. Am J Public Health 71:85–87, 1981

Boyle CA, Decoufle P, O'Brien TR: Long-term health consequences of military service in Vietnam. Epidemiol Rev 11:1–27, 1989

Branscomb LP: Dissociation in combat-related posttraumatic stress disorder. Dissociation 4:13–20, 1991

Bremner JD, Southwick SM, Brett E, et al: Dissociation and PTSD in Vietnam combat veterans. Am J Psychiatry 149:328–333, 1992

Bremner JD, Southwick SM, Johnson DR, et al: Childhood physical abuse in combat-related posttraumatic stress disorder. Am J Psychiatry 150:133–136, 1993a

Bremner JD, Davis M, Southwick SM, et al: Neurobiology of posttraumatic stress disorder, in American Psychiatric Press Review of Psychiatry, Vol 12. Edited by Oldham JM, Riba MB, Tasman A. Washington, DC, American Psychiatric Press, 1993b, pp 183–204

Bremner JD, Steinberg M, Southwick SM, et al: Use of the Structured Clinical Interview for DSM-IV-Dissociative Disorders for systematic assessment of dissociative symptoms in posttraumatic stress disorder. Am J Psychiatry 150:1011–1014, 1993c

Bremner JD, Southwick SM, Darnell A, et al: The longitudinal course of posttraumatic stress disorder in Vietnam combat veterans: development, longitudinal course, and relationship to alcohol and substance abuse. Arch Gen Psychiatry (in press)

Breslau N, Davis GC: Posttraumatic stress disorder: the stressor criterion. J Nerv Ment Dis 175:255–264, 1987a

Breslau N, Davis GC: Posttraumatic stress disorder: the etiologic specificity of wartime stressors. Am J Psychiatry 144:578–583, 1987b

Breslau N, Davis GC: Posttraumatic stress disorder in an urban population of young adults: risk factors for chronicity. Am J Psychiatry 49:671–675, 1992

Breslau N, Davis GC, Andreski P, et al: Traumatic events and posttraumatic stress disorder in an urban population of young adults. Arch Gen Psychiatry 48:216–222, 1991

Brett E, Spitzer RL, Williams JBW: DSM-III-R criteria for posttraumatic stress disorder. Am J Psychiatry 145:1232–1236, 1988

Cadoret RJ, Winokur G, Dorzab J, et al: Depressive disease: life events and onset of illness. Arch Gen Psychiatry 26:133–136, 1972

Card JJ: Lives After Vietnam: The Personal Impact of Military Service. Lexington, MA, Heath, 1983

Card JJ: Epidemiology of PTSD in a national cohort of Vietnam veterans. J Clin Psychol 43:6–17, 1987

Cardeña E, Spiegel D: Dissociative reactions to the San Francisco Bay Area earthquake of 1989. Am J Psychiatry 150:474–478, 1993

Carlson EB, Rosser-Hogan R: Trauma experiences, posttraumatic stress, dissociation, and depression in Cambodian refugees. Am J Psychiatry 148:1548–1552, 1991

Carmen EH, Riekker PP, Mills T: Victims of violence and psychiatric illness. Am J Psychiatry 141:378–383, 1984

Carroll EM, Rueger DB, Foy DW, et al: Vietnam combat veterans with posttraumatic stress disorder: analysis of marital and cohabiting adjustment. J Abnorm Psychol 94:329–337, 1985

Centers for Disease Control: The Centers for Disease Control Vietnam Experiences Study: health status of Vietnam veterans, I: psychosocial characteristics. JAMA 259:2701–2707, 1988a

Centers for Disease Control: The Centers for Disease Control Vietnam Experiences Study: health status of Vietnam veterans, II: physical health. JAMA 259:2708–2714, 1988b

Chemtob CM, Bauer GB, Neller G: Posttraumatic stress disorder among Special Forces Vietnam veterans. Mil Med 155:16–20, 1990

Chrousos GP, Gold PW: The concepts of stress and stress system disorders. JAMA 267:1244–1252, 1992

Chu JA, Dill DL: Dissociative symptoms in relation to childhood physical and sexual abuse. Am J Psychiatry 147:887–892, 1990

Coleman JC, Burcher JN, Carson RC: Abnormal Psychology and Modern Life, 6th Edition. Blenview, IL, Scott Foresman, 1980

Davidson J, Swartz M, Storck M, et al: A diagnostic and family study of posttraumatic stress disorder. Am J Psychiatry 142:90–93, 1985

Davidson J, Smith R, Kudler HS: Familial psychiatric illness in chronic posttraumatic stress disorder. Compr Psychiatry 30:339–345, 1989

Eaton WW, Sigal JJ, Weinfeld M: Impairment in holocaust survivors after 33 years: data from an unbiased community sample. Am J Psychiatry 139:773–777, 1982

Egendorf A, Kaduschin C, Laufer RS, et al: Legacies of Vietnam: Comparative Adjustment of Veterans and Their Peers. Washington, DC, Government Printing Office, 1981

Elder GH, Clipp EC: Wartime losses and social bonding: influences across 40 years in men's lives. Psychiatry 51:177–198, 1988

Emery VO, Emery PE, Shama DK, et al: Predisposing variables in PTSD patients. Journal of Traumatic Stress 4:325–343, 1991

Escobar JI, Randolph EY, Guadalupe P, et al: Post-traumatic stress disorder in Hispanic Vietnam veterans: clinical phenomenology and sociocultural characteristics. J Nerv Ment Dis 171:585–596, 1983

Faustman WO, White PA: Diagnostic and psychopharmacological treatment characteristics of 536 inpatients with posttraumatic stress disorder. J Nerv Ment Dis 177:154–159, 1989

Figley CR: Psychological adjustment among Vietnam veterans: an overview of the research, in Stress Disorders Among Vietnam Veterans. Edited by Figley CR. New York, Brunner/Mazel, 1978, pp 57–70

Finkelhor D, Araji S, Baron L, et al: A Sourcebook on Child Sexual Abuse. Beverly Hills, CA, Sage, 1986

Fontana A, Rosenheck R: A causal model of the etiology of war-related PTSD. Journal of Traumatic Stress (in press)

Foy DW, Card JJ: Combat-related posttraumatic stress disorder etiology: replicated findings in a national sample of Vietnam-era men. J Clin Psychol 43:28–31, 1987

Foy DW, Rueger DB, Sipprelle RC, et al: Etiology of posttraumatic stress disorder in Vietnam veterans: analysis of premilitary, military, and combat exposure influences. J Consult Clin Psychol 52:79–87, 1984

Foy DW, Carroll EM, Donahoe CP Jr: Etiological factors in the development of PTSD in clinical samples of Vietnam combat veterans. J Clin Psychol 43:17–27, 1987

Freud S, Ferenczi S, Abraham K, et al: Psychoanalysis and the War Neurosis. New York, International Psychoanalytic Press, 1921

Frye J, Stockton RA: Discriminant analysis of posttraumatic stress disorder among a group of Vietnam combat veterans. Am J Psychiatry 139:52–56, 1982

Gallers J, Foy DW, Donohoe CP, et al: Posttraumatic stress disorder in Vietnam combat veterans: effects of traumatic violence exposure and military adjustment. J Traum Stress 1:181–192, 1988

Ghaziuddin M, Ghaziuddin N, Stein GS: Life events and the recurrence of depression. Can J Psychiatry 35:239–242, 1990

Gleser GC, Green BL, Winget CN: Prolonged Psychosocial Effects of Disaster. New York, Academic Press, 1981

Goldberg J, True WR, Eisen SA, et al: A twin study of the effects of the Vietnam war on posttraumatic stress disorder. JAMA 263:1227–1232, 1990

Green BL, Grace MC, Gleser GC: Identifying survivors at risk: long-term impairment following the Beverly Hills Supper Club fire. J Consult Clin Psychol 53:672–678, 1985

Green BL, Lindy JD, Grace MC, et al: Multiple diagnosis in posttraumatic stress disorder: the role of war stressors. J Nerv Ment Dis 177:329–335, 1989

Green BL, Grace MC, Lindy JD, et al: Race differences in response to combat stress. J Traum Stress 3:379–393, 1990a

Green BL, Grace MC, Lindy JD, et al: Risk factors for PTSD and other diagnoses in a general sample of Vietnam veterans. Am J Psychiatry 147:729–733, 1990b

Green BL, Lindy JD, Grace MC, et al: Chronic posttraumatic stress disorder and diagnostic comorbidity in a disaster sample. J Nerv Ment Dis 180:760–766, 1992

Green MA, Berlin MA: Five psychosocial variables related to the existence of posttraumatic stress disorder symptoms. J Clin Psychol 43:643–649, 1987

Hastings TJ: The Stanford-Terman study revisited: postwar emotional health of World War II veterans. Military Psychology 3:201–214, 1991

Helzer JE, Robins LN, Davis DH: Depressive disorders in Vietnam returnees. J Nerv Ment Dis 163:177–185, 1976

Helzer JE, Robins LN, Wish E, et al: Depression in Vietnam veterans and civilian controls. Am J Psychiatry 136:526–529, 1979

Helzer JE, Robins LN, McEvoy L: Post-traumatic stress disorder in the general population: findings of the epidemiologic catchment area survey. N Engl J Med 317:1630–1634, 1987

Henderson JL, Moore M: The psychoneurosis of war. N Engl J Med 230:274–278, 1944

Herman J, Russell D, Trocki K: Long-term effects of incestuous abuse in childhood. Am J Psychiatry 143:1293–1296, 1986

Keane TM, Fairbank JA: Survey analysis of combat-related stress disorders in Vietnam veterans. Am J Psychiatry 140:348–350, 1983

Keane TM, Scott WO, Chavoya GA, et al: Social support in Vietnam veterans with posttraumatic stress disorder: a comparative analysis. J Consult Clin Psychol 53:95–102, 1985

Keane TM, Caddell JM, Taylor KL: Mississippi Scale for Combat-Related Post-Traumatic Stress Disorder: three studies in reliability and validity. J Consult Clin Psychol 56:85–90, 1988

Kilpatrick DG, Best CL, Veronen LJ, et al: Mental health correlates of criminal victimization: a random community survey. J Consult Clin Psychol 53:866–873, 1985

Kulka RA, Schlenger WE, Fairbank JA, et al: National Vietnam Veterans Readjustment Study: Tables of Findings and Technical Appendices. New York, Brunner/Mazel, 1990

Lazarus RS: Thoughts on the relation between emotion and cognition, in Approaches to Emotion. Edited by Scherer KR, Ekman P. Hillsdale, NJ, Erlbaum, 1984, pp 247–158

Laufer RS, Brett E, Gallops MS: Dimensions of posttraumatic stress disorder among Vietnam veterans. J Nerv Ment Dis 173:538–545, 1985a

Laufer RS, Brett E, Gallops MS: Symptom patterns associated with post-traumatic stress disorder among Vietnam veterans exposed to war trauma. Am J Psychiatry 142:1304–1311, 1985b

Loewenstein R, Putnam F: A comparison study of dissociative symptoms in patients with complex partial seizures, MPD, and PTSD. Dissociation 1:17–23, 1988

March JS: What constitutes a stressor? The "Criterion A" issue, in Post-traumatic Stress Disorder: DSM-IV and Beyond. Edited by Davidson JRT, Foa EB. Washington, DC, American Psychiatric Press, 1993, pp 37–54

McFarlane AC: The aetiology of posttraumatic stress disorders following a natural disaster. Br J Psychiatry 152:116–121, 1988a

McFarlane AC: The longitudinal course of posttraumatic morbidity: the range of outcomes and their predictors. J Nerv Ment Dis 176:30–39, 1988b

Nace EP, O'Brien CP, Mintz J, et al: Adjustment among Vietnam veteran drug users two years post service, in Stress Disorders Among Vietnam Veterans. Edited by Figley CR. New York, Brunner/Mazel, 1978

Nemiah JC: Janet redivivus: the centenary of l'Automatisme Psychologique. Am J Psychiatry 146:1527–1530, 1989

Nefzger MD: Follow-up studies of World War II and Korean war prisoners; I: study plan and mortality findings. Am J Epidemiol 91:123–138, 1970

Norris FH: Epidemiology of trauma: frequency and impact of different potentially traumatic events on different demographic groups. J Consult Clin Psychol 60:409–418, 1992

Paykel ES, Prusoff BA, Myers JK: Suicide attempts and recent life events: a controlled comparison. Arch Gen Psychiatry 32:327–333, 1975

Penk WE, Robinowitz R, Roberts WR, et al: Adjustment differences among male substance abusers varying in degree of combat experience in Vietnam. J Consult Clin Psychol 49:426–437, 1981

Penk WE, Robinowitz R, Black J, et al: Ethnicity: posttraumatic stress disorder (PTSD) differences among black, white, and Hispanic veterans who differ in degrees of exposure to combat in Vietnam. J Clin Psychol 45:729–735, 1989

Pynoos RS, Frederick C, Nader K, et al: Life threat and posttraumatic stress in school-age children. Arch Gen Psychiatry 44:1057–1063, 1987

Resnick HS, Foy DW, Donahoe CP, et al: Antisocial behavior and posttraumatic stress disorder in Vietnam veterans. J Clin Psychol 45:861–866, 1989

Resnick HS, Kilpatrick DG, Best CL, et al: Vulnerability-stress factors in the development of posttraumatic stress disorder. J Nerv Ment Dis 180:424–430, 1992

Rosenheck R: Impact of posttraumatic stress disorder of World War II on the next generation. J Nerv Ment Dis 174:319–327, 1986

Rosenheck R, Nathan P: Secondary traumatization in children of Vietnam veterans. Hosp Community Psychiatry 36:538–539, 1985

Russell D: The Secret Trauma: Incest in the Lives of Girls and Women. New York, Basic Books, 1986

Schnurr PP, Friedman MJ, Rosenberg SD: Preliminary MMPI scores as predictors of combat related PTSD symptoms. Am J Psychiatry 150:479–483, 1993

Selye H: The Stress of Life. New York, McGraw-Hill, 1956

Sierles FS, Chen JJ, McFarland RE, et al: Posttraumatic stress disorder and concurrent psychiatric illness: a preliminary report. Am J Psychiatry 140:1177–1179, 1983

Solkoff N, Gray P, Keill S: Which Vietnam veterans develop posttraumatic stress disorders? J Clin Psychol 42:687–698, 1986

Solomon Z, Mikulincer M, Jakob BR: Exposure to recurrent combat stress: combat stress reactions among Israeli soldiers in the Lebanon War. Psychol Med 17:433–440, 1987a

Solomon Z, Garb R, Bleich A, et al: Reactivation of combat-related posttraumatic stress disorder. Am J Psychiatry 144:51–55, 1987b

Southwick SM, Morgan A, Nagy LM, et al: Trauma related symptomatology in Desert Storm veterans: a preliminary report. Am J Psychiatry 150:1524–1528, 1993

Speed N, Engdahl B, Schwartz J, et al: Posttraumatic stress disorder as a consequence of the POW experience. J Nerv Ment Dis 177:147–153, 1989

Spiegel D, Cardeña E: Disintegrated experience: the dissociative disorders revisited. J Abnorm Psych 100:366–378, 1991

Spiegel D, Hunt T, Dondershine HE: Dissociation and hypnotizability in posttraumatic stress disorder. Am J Psychiatry 145:301–305, 1988

Steinberg M, Rounsaville B, Cicchetti DV: The Structured Clinical Interview for DSM-III-R Dissociative Disorders: preliminary report on a new diagnostic instrument. Am J Psychiatry 147:76–82, 1990

Stutman RK, Bliss EL: Posttraumatic stress disorder, hypnotizability, and imagery. Am J Psychiatry 142:741–743, 1985

Swett C, Surrey J, Cohen C: Sexual and physical abuse histories and psychiatric symptoms among male psychiatric outpatients. Am J Psychiatry 147:632–636, 1990

Torrie A: Psychosomatic casualties in the Middle East. Lancet 29:139–143, 1944

True WR, Goldberg J, Eisen SA: Stress symptomatology among Vietnam veterans: analysis of the Veterans Administration survey of veterans, II. Am J Epidemiol 128:85–92, 1988

Ursano RJ: The Vietnam era prisoner of war: precaptivity personality and the development of psychiatric illness. Am J Psychiatry 138:315–318, 1981

Ursano RJ, Boydstun JA, Wheatley RD: Psychiatric illness in U.S. Air Force Vietnam prisoners of war: a five-year follow-up. Am J Psychiatry 138:310–314, 1981

van der Kolk BA, van der Hart O: Pierre Janet and the breakdown of adaptation in psychological trauma. Am J Psychiatry 146:1530–1540, 1989

Vinokur A, Caplan RD, Williams CC: Effects of recent and past stress on mental health: coping with unemployment among Vietnam veterans and nonveterans. Journal of Applied and Social Psychology 17:710–730, 1987

Warheit GJ: Life events, coping, stress, and depressive symptomatology. Am J Psychiatry 136:502–507, 1979

Wolfe J, Brown PJ, Bucsela ML: Symptom responses of female Vietnam veterans to Operation Desert Storm. Am J Psychiatry 149:676–680, 1992

Worthington ER: Post-service adjustment and Vietnam era veterans. Mil Med 142:865–866, 1977

Worthington ER: Demographic and preservice variables as predictors of post-military service adjustment, in Stress Disorders Among Vietnam Veterans. Edited by Figley CR. New York, Brunner/Mazel, 1978, pp 173–187

Wyatt GE, Guthrie D, Notgrass CM: Differential effects of women's child sexual abuse and subsequent sexual revictimization. J Consult Clin Psychol 60:167–173, 1992

Yager J: Personal violence in infantry combat. Arch Gen Psychiatry 32:257–261, 1975

Yager T, Laufer R, Gallops M: Some problems associated with war experience in men of the Vietnam generation. Arch Gen Psychiatry 41:327–333, 1984

Yehuda R, Southwick SM, Giller EL: Exposure to atrocities and severity of chronic posttraumatic stress disorder in Vietnam combat veterans. Am J Psychiatry 149:333–336, 1992

Chapter 7

Stress of Bereavement and Consequent Psychiatric Illness

Kathleen Kim, M.D., M.P.H., and
Selby Jacobs, M.D., M.P.H.

BEREAVEMENT AS A MODEL FOR THE RELATIONSHIP BETWEEN STRESS AND PSYCHIATRIC STATE

The findings from several hundred studies support the hypothesis that life stressors of all types place individuals at greater risk for a variety of physical and mental disorders (Elliott and Eisdorfer 1982). According to stress researchers, bereavement is the most severe stressor of adult life (Holmes and Rahe 1967), and a significant minority of adults experience adverse consequences: an increase in overall mortality (Helsing et al. 1981; Rees and Lutkins 1967); an increase in the relative risk of death from cardiovascular disease (Engel 1971), accidents, and some infectious diseases (Helsing et al. 1982) in widowers; an increase in the relative risk of death from cirrhosis in widows (Helsing et al. 1982); and an increased risk of suicidal gestures (Birtchnell 1970) and suicide following spousal and parental deaths (MacMahon and Pugh 1965; Murphy et al. 1979; Stein and Susser 1969).

We believe that bereavement serves as an ideal model for examining the relationship between a significant stressor and mental health and the risk factors that distinguish those who develop psychiatric complications from those who do not. This chapter consists of four sections. The literature on normal and pathologic grief is reviewed in the first section. The differential diagnosis of psychiatric disorders during bereavement is described in the second section. Empirical data on the psychiatric complications and risk factors that lead to these complications are presented in the third section. Finally, some clinical implications of complicated bereavement are discussed in the fourth section.

Phases of Normal Grief

There are four phases of normal grief: emotional numbing and disbelief, separation distress, mourning, and recovery. Certain manifestations predominate in each phase, and the phases can overlap during the course of bereavement.

The initial phase of grief is characterized by emotional numbing or disbelief. It lasts from a few hours to several days (usually 2–5 days but no longer than 2 weeks). Emotional numbing and disbelief are symptoms of avoidance and are often seen in the circumstances of a sudden loss. In addition, they may be accompanied by intrusive symptoms, such as horrific images and nightmares, which are associated with traumatic distress. Traumatic distress is conspicuous when a loss is caused by an accident or natural disaster. It represents an injury to the person's sense of well-being and his or her assumption of living in a safe, predictable world.

The second phase of grief is separation distress. Among adults, separation distress includes yearning for the lost person, being preoccupied with the deceased, crying, having episodes associated with a perceptual set for the lost person (dreams, tactile or visual illusions, hallucinations in some cases), and searching for the person (seeking out places and things identified with the deceased). The yearning is intrusive, episodic, and time limited (20–30 minutes); Lindemann (1944) named the phenomenon the pang of grief. Since the search for the lost person is fruitless, it culminates in acute separation distress, with peak intensity 6–8 weeks after the loss. Eventually, the search is abandoned, and the irrevocability of the loss is accepted emotionally and cognitively. As a result, the separation distress subsides.

The third phase of grief is the mourning process. During this phase, the bereaved person begins to remember the deceased in new and different ways. The bereaved repeatedly reviews the lost relationship with sad, nostalgic, and sometimes angry and guilty feelings (Freud 1917/1962; Raphael 1983). The mourning process is associated with depressive symptoms, such as sorrow, dysphoria, despair, and neurovegetative symptoms. The depressive symptoms reach peak intensity later than do separation distress symptoms.

The fourth phase of grief is recovery. Recovery involves a cognitive process of accepting the new status and mastering new roles. Acute changes in status may be associated with emotional and physiologic arousal and may cause excess mortality due to cardiovascular disease among widowers. Longer term changes may be associated with suicide, as the risk of suicide extends for several years after a loss (MacMahon and Pugh 1965).

The duration of normal grief is subject to debate. Most mental health researchers believe that separation distress and the mourning process begin to diminish 4–6 months after the loss (Windholz et al. 1985). Social scientists disagree; they believe that the emotional distress of bereavement extends beyond the first 6 months and begins to attenuate sometime during the first year of bereavement (Barrett and Schneweis 1980; Silverman 1986). Social adjustment to widowhood commences after cognitive acceptance of the loss when the emotional distress subsides in intensity. The adjustment may extend over several years (Silverman 1986).

Pathologic Grief

Pathologic grief is distinguished from normal grief by the nature, duration, and severity of symptoms. Although the concept of pathologic grief has been well described, there was no consensus on the diagnostic criteria of the syndrome until recently (Raphael and Middleton 1990).

In his classic work, "Mourning and Melancholia," Freud (1917/1962) described the differences between the two phenomena. Mourning was distinguished by painful dejection, cessation of interest in the outside world, loss of the capacity to love, and inhibition of activity. Melancholia was distinguished by a disturbance of self-esteem. Freud hypothesized that the nature of the relationship with the deceased was a crucial determinant of the survivor's adjustment to loss. If the survivor's relationship to the deceased was narcissistic or ambivalent, the attributes of the lost person were psychologically introjected. Anger at the deceased for dying was directed inwardly by the survivor, and the survivor would become depressed. Freud used the term *pathological mourning* to describe this psychodynamic process.

Deutsch (1937) was the first to suggest that the absence of grief was pathologic. She described four patients who did not exhibit normal manifestations of grief. Instead, they expressed grief through neurotic symptoms and/or narcissistic or schizoid character traits.

In separate articles, Lindemann (1944) and Adler (1943) described the presentation of survivors of the November 1942 Coconut Grove nightclub fire in Boston, Massachusetts, and developed typologies based on the symptoms of these survivors. Lindemann developed a typology of morbid grief reactions: delayed grief (the manifestations of grief were delayed for 2 or more weeks) and nine clinical presentations of distorted grief (the expression of grief in other than separation distress symptoms). Adler, whose work was largely ignored until the early 1970s, was the first to recognize the clinically traumatic aspects of the Coconut Grove fire. She attributed the victims' neuropsychiatric complications to the losses as well as the trauma of the fire. Adler characterized the complications of bereavement as anxiety neuroses, including symptoms similar to posttraumatic stress disorder (PTSD).

Bowlby and Parkes used separation distress as a paradigm to characterize child and adult bereavement (Bowlby 1973; Bowlby and Parkes 1970); this paradigm was based on Darwin's (1872) *The Expression of the Emotions in Man and Animals.* In the book, Darwin described the loss reaction in animals and its similarity to grief in humans. Bowlby and Parkes believed that searching (seeking out places and things identified with the deceased) was as integral a part of human grief as it was in animals. They viewed separation anxiety as a basic human response independent of sexual and self-protective drives, which promoted survival in social animals.

After investigating several hypotheses, Bowlby (1980) described two categories of pathologic grief: chronic mourning (prolonged and severe) and absent grief with persistent anger and self-reproach associated with depression. Bowlby's formulations were based on cognitive theory. He hypothesized that the bereaved person may have negative cognitive biases about attachment figures and, as a consequence, may exhibit behaviors that can become maladaptive.

Based on direct observational studies, Parkes and Weiss (1983) created a typology that identified characteristics of the death and characteristics of the relationship with the deceased as part of the clinical syndrome of pathologic grief. The typology included 1) unanticipated grief with feelings of denial, self-reproach, and despair; 2) conflicted grief with grief being delayed or absent secondary to ambivalent feelings toward the deceased; and 3) chronic grief secondary to a dependent relationship with the deceased because of antecedent insecurity.

Using a cognitive perspective, Horowitz (1976) incorporated traumatic distress as a main component of the emotional response of bereavement. He integrated the idea of emotional trauma with separation distress and developed an assessment form, the Impact of Event Scale (Horowitz et al. 1979). By combining trauma with loss, Horowitz made the implicit assumption that all losses are traumatic. More recent studies indicate that traumatic distress and separation anxiety are independent but linked dimensions of grief (Nader et al. 1990; Pynoos et al. 1987). Horowitz viewed pathologic grief as a prolongation or intensification of formerly "controlled" ego states (i.e., ego states that had been held in check by the relationship with the deceased). These ego states are either frighteningly sad or enraged or deflated states that reflect underlying borderline or narcissistic personality traits (Horowitz et al. 1980).

In the early 1970s, Clayton renewed interest in the distinction between mourning and the depressions of bereavement (Clayton et al. 1971, 1974). She and her colleagues found that 45% of acutely bereaved spouses developed depressive syndromes sometime during the first year of bereavement (Bornstein et al. 1973). They were the first to use structured assessments of depression in their studies. Although most of these depressions were transient and subsided spontaneously, 17% of the sample remained depressed throughout the entire first year of bereavement. The evolution of symptoms was similar to melancholic depression (Clayton and Darvish 1979).

Similar to Clayton's work, more recent studies have begun to document the risk of anxiety disorders during acute bereavement (Jacobs et al. 1990; Zisook et al. 1990). These anxiety syndromes include panic disorder and generalized anxiety disorder (GAD). Both of these disorders can occur independently from the depressions of bereavement, particularly panic disorder (Jacobs et al. 1990).

In 1990, Raphael and Middleton developed consensus criteria for the diagnosis of pathologic grief. According to the criteria, there are three variants of pathologic grief: 1) delayed or absent grief, 2) inhibited grief, and 3) chronic grief (see Table 7–1 in next section). The consensus criteria assume a normal progression of grief over time (described in the subsection on the normal phases of grief). Although these criteria have not been tested for consistency in family history, utility for prognosis, biological correlates, concurrent validity with respect to functional impairment, disability, and risk for subsequent morbidity and mortality, they do represent the consensus of bereavement experts. They are the best working diagnostic criteria available.

Delayed grief is defined as delayed manifestations of grief for 2 or more weeks. If the delay becomes prolonged, it is absent grief. The bereaved may appear to be acting as though nothing has happened, or emotional distress may appear but after a substantial time. In particular, there is a lack of separation distress symptoms. A general depressive response may be delayed or absent. Alternatively, the delay or absence may be related to the presence of other phenomena, such as PTSD.

Inhibited grief is defined as the attenuation of the typical manifestations of separation distress and the exaggeration of ancillary symptomatology, such as distorted grief. Distorted grief is marked by somatic symptoms; identification symptoms; overt hostility; affective blunting (related to hostility); self-reproach; and self-destructive, overactive, socially withdrawn, or vicarious caregiver behavior. Depressive or anxious symptoms may be prominent in distorted grief.

Chronic grief is defined as intense manifestations of separation distress that do not diminish throughout the first year of bereavement and beyond. The bereaved person fails to demonstrate a phasic response with progression through the bereavement process. The person may become locked into any one of grief's dimensions and does not progress into further areas. Grief continues with an intensity that is normally expected in the first months of the acute phase after the loss. The high level of intensity carries on for 6 months or more and may be present for 2 or more years later.

DIFFERENTIAL DIAGNOSIS OF PSYCHIATRIC DISORDERS DURING ACUTE BEREAVEMENT

In this section, we summarize guidelines for distinguishing normal grief symptoms from the psychiatric complications of bereavement. Although most laypersons, clergy, primary care physicians, and some mental health professionals believe that emotional distress is a necessary part of grief (Wortman and Silver 1989), it is important to distinguish the symptoms of normal grief from the syndromes of pathologic grief and psychiatric disorders. An accurate diagnosis can guide interventions for appropriate treatment, which can alleviate morbidity and, in some cases, prevent mortality.

Normal Grief Versus Pathologic Grief

Delayed grief is often associated with traumatic or sudden, unexpected deaths (Parkes and Weiss 1983); severe symptomatology of other types, such as depressive symptoms and pain syndromes; or no other signs of disturbance. Those with delayed grief often present to psychiatrists late in the course of bereavement with chronic grief syndrome (Kim and Jacobs 1991) or major depression (Kim and Jacobs 1991; Parkes and Weiss 1983). Jacobs (1993) estimated that 10%–15% of patients present with delayed grief and usually in the context of a traumatic loss. Delayed grief is distinguished from normal grief by a 2-week or more delay of separation distress symptoms, by the severity of symptoms, and by the abnormal progression of grief (see summary and Table 7–1).

Table 7–1. Differential diagnosis of normal and pathologic grief

Criterion	Normal	Delayed/absent	Severe	Inhibited	Chronic
Onset of separation distress	Within 2 weeks	Delayed more than 2 weeks	Immediate, sometimes delayed	Within 2 weeks	Sometimes delayed
Numbness, disbelief	Transient, usually a few days	Severe, persistent, or absent	Severe or transient	Transient	Sometimes severe, persistent
Separation distress	Transient, peaks usually in 4–6 weeks	Absent	Severe, fear of losing control	Attenuated, sometimes absent	Sometimes severe
Distorted symptoms	Absent or minimal			Severe	Sometimes prominent
Depressive symptoms	Transient, peak usually in 4–6 months	Sometimes severe		Sometimes severe	Usually severe
Anxiety symptoms	Transient		Usually severe	Sometimes severe	Sometimes severe
Evolution of grief or recovery	Acceptance, some improvement by 1 year	Prolonged	Prolonged	Prolonged	Prolonged
Psychiatric comorbidity	Rare	High risk of MDD	High risk of MDD and AD	Risk of MDD	High risk of MDD and AD

Note. MDD = major depressive disorder; AD = anxiety disorder.

Absent grief is characterized by the lack of any symptoms of distress for an extended period of time following the loss (6 months to a year). Jacobs (1993) estimated that 5% of patients have absent grief and that these patients are at higher risk for major depression. Absent grief is distinguished from normal grief by the absence of any manifestations of grief.

Inhibited grief is characterized by the attenuation of the typical manifestations of separation distress and the exaggeration of distorted grief. Distorted grief is marked by somatic symptoms, identification symptoms, and self-reproach, among other symptoms. Jacobs (1993) estimated that 5%–10% of patients present with inhibited grief; they usually present with distorted grief symptoms and on anniversaries of the loss. Inhibited grief is distinguished from normal grief by the diminution of typical separation distress symptoms, by distorted grief, and by the abnormal progression of grief.

Several researchers consider severe grief another variant of pathologic grief. It is characterized by the exaggeration of the manifestations of normal separation distress. Bereaved persons with severe grief are at higher risk for developing depressive and anxiety disorders (Bornstein et al. 1973; Jacobs et al. 1989; Zisook and DeVaul 1983). There are no estimates of the occurrence of severe grief. Severe grief is differentiated from normal grief by the severity of symptoms and by the abnormal progression of grief.

Chronic grief implies a failure of the normal progression of grief; the bereaved does not accept the loss, or the symptoms do not attenuate with time. In some cases, separation distress worsens at the first anniversary of the loss (Cleiren 1991; Sanders 1989). Jacobs (1993) reported that chronic grief is the most common variation of pathologic grief. Chronic grief is differentiated from normal grief by the prolonged severity of symptoms and by the abnormal progression of grief.

Normal Depressive Symptoms Versus Major Depressive Episode

Since the early 1970s, many researchers have examined the distinction between mourning and the depressions of bereavement.

Depressive syndromes are observed in up to 45% of bereaved persons (Bornstein et al. 1973; Jacobs et al. 1989; Zisook and Shuchter 1991), but most of these syndromes (80%) are transient and resolve spontaneously in 6 months or less. The minority (20%) are persistent, impair functioning, and are unremitting. Major depression is distinguished from normal depressive symptoms of grief by pervasive disturbance of self-esteem (Bornstein et al. 1973; Freud 1917/1962; Parkes 1972), by marked psychomotor retardation (Bornstein et al. 1973; Clayton et al. 1974), and by suicidal gestures (Bornstein et al. 1973; Clayton et al. 1974).

The normal depressive symptoms of bereavement last for several weeks. In the first 6 months of bereavement, several symptoms can be used as distinguishing criteria to diagnose a major depression. These include psychotic symptoms, guilt, psychomotor retardation, severe impairment in functioning, and suicidal ideation or attempts (Jacobs 1993).

It has been recommended that the standard DSM-III-R (American Psychiatric Association 1987) criteria be used to diagnose major depression after an individual has experienced 6 months of bereavement (Jacobs 1993). If anhedonia, self-depreciation, anger, and increased alcohol use persist and are more prominent later in the course of bereavement, the individual is more likely to have a major depression (Blanchard et al. 1976; Clayton and Darvish 1979).

The persistence of depressive mood and neurovegetative symptoms beyond 1 year is unusual for normal grief (Blanchard et al. 1976; Clayton and Darvish 1979). The differential diagnosis of normal depressive symptoms and major depressive episode is summarized in Table 7–2.

Normal Anxiety Symptoms Versus Anxiety Disorder

Less is known about the incidence and course of anxiety symptoms during bereavement. Currently, there are no distinctive symptoms that distinguish normal anxiety symptoms from anxiety disorders in the bereaved. For example, the fear of losing control is a nonspecific symptom of anxiety disorders and pathologic grief. It can indicate that separation distress is severe or that

Table 7–2. Differential diagnosis of the depressive symptoms of bereavement and major depressive disorder superimposed on bereavement

	Bereavement	Depression
Symptomatic criteria		
Self-esteem	Focused feeling of guilt; feeling useless; "the world is poor and empty"	Pervasive and unrealistic feeling of guilt; feeling worthless; "it's the ego itself that is poor and empty"
Psychomotor disturbance	Agitation is seen; retardation seldom, if ever	Agitation and retardation
Suicidal gestures	Rare, although risk is higher	Common
Hallucinations and delusions	Focused on deceased	Congruent with depression, pessimism, and poor self-esteem
Duration and timing of depressive symptoms	Early syndromes common, mostly transient; neurovegetative symptoms usually transient	Persistent
Psychosocial stress	Loss	Persistent stress may be associated with depression
Social and occupational functioning	Transient, minor impairment	Impairment by time of consultation
Personal and family history		
Sex ratio	Female = Male	Female > Male
History of depression	Common	Common
Family history of depression	?	Common

the bereaved is experiencing GAD or panic disorder (Clayton et al. 1971).

The diagnosis of an anxiety disorder is based primarily on the degree to which anxiety symptoms impair a bereaved person's ability to function. Anxiety symptoms are considered severe when the individual cannot manage emotional and instrumental tasks, take responsibility for self-care, or fulfill parental or occupational roles.

PTSD is commonly associated with traumatic distress and delayed grief. The dissociative processes of PTSD include severe emotional numbing and disbelief. However, the intrusive symptoms (e.g., flashbacks) and increased arousal of PTSD are not associated with normal grief. PTSD is differentiated from normal anxiety symptoms by intrusive symptoms, by hypervigilance, and by persistent autonomic arousal.

PSYCHIATRIC COMPLICATIONS OF BEREAVEMENT

In contrast to past bereavement studies, recent studies have adopted an atheoretical or nonetiological model of psychiatric disorders, as exemplified by DSM-III-R. These studies have avoided conceptual models of pathologic grief and focused on the descriptive quantification of symptoms. They have used diagnostic interview schedules or dimensional distress scales to assess psychiatric status in bereaved persons.

Based on data from the Structured Clinical Interview for DSM-III (Spitzer et al. 1985), acutely bereaved spouses were found to be at higher risk for depressions and anxiety disorders than the general population (Jacobs et al. 1989, 1990). In a prospective community sample, conjugal bereavement was associated with an increased risk of major depressive episode and dysphoria (Bruce et al. 1990). Two studies have reported moderately high correlations among dimensional measures of unresolved grief, depression, and anxiety (Jacobs 1987; Zisook and DeVaul 1983). These findings indicate the concurrence of symptoms of these disorders but do not distinguish whether the symptoms of pathologic grief are similar or identical to other psychiatric disorders.

The rate of psychiatric complications of bereavement is dependent on the definition of adverse outcome: For pathologic grief, the rate range is 4%–34% (Maddison and Viola 1968; Parkes and Weiss 1983; Zisook and DeVaul 1983); for major depression, the rate range is 17%–31% (Bornstein et al. 1973; Bruce et al. 1990; Jacobs et al. 1989); for panic disorder, the rate is 13% (Jacobs et al. 1990); and for GAD, the rate is 39% (Jacobs et al. 1990). The rate of comorbidity is significant, with more than half of acutely bereaved spouses suffering from two disorders (Jacobs and Kim 1990; Kim and Jacobs 1991). The variation in rates of disorders is probably due to differences in study design, sample sizes and characteristics, and changes in populations over time (e.g., increases in rates of depression).

Pathologic Grief and Its Relationship to Other Psychiatric Disorders

We conducted a clinical study (Kim and Jacobs 1991) to elucidate pathologic grief and its relationship to major depression and anxiety disorders (i.e., panic disorder and GAD). At the time of the study, there were no standardized criteria for pathologic grief, so we defined explicit diagnostic criteria and used them to address three main questions: Is pathologic grief isomorphic (i.e., similar in form) with depression? Is pathologic grief isomorphic with anxiety disorders? What is the relationship between the diagnosis of pathologic grief and dimensional screening measures of emotional distress?

Methods. The sample was collected by referral from a trained research interviewer who was testing telephone screening procedures for depression and anxiety disorders. Candidates for participation were identified through systematic screening of death certificates in the Office of Vital Statistics for a medium-sized metropolitan area. When the interviewer encountered a bereaved spouse who seemed depressed or anxious or appeared to be having difficulty with grief, the interviewer invited the spouse to take part in a psychiatric interview. Of 76 bereaved persons screened, 25 widows and widowers agreed to participate. All of the sample had been bereaved for longer than 6 months, and 13

(52%) had passed the first anniversary of the loss. This pilot sample was not random. The bereaved spouses who feared a psychiatric interview were likely to decline, and those who denied emotional distress subsequent to the loss were less likely to be identified as possible participants. Data on the nonparticipants were not available to test these assumptions.

During the telephone interview, the research interviewer collected data on several self-report measures of emotional distress, including 1) the 20-item Center for Epidemiologic Studies— Depression (CES-D) Scale (Comstock and Helsing 1976; Weissman et al. 1979), 2) the 10-item Psychiatric Epidemiology Research Instrument (PERI) anxiety scale (Dohrenwend et al. 1980), 3) measures of separation distress (12 items) and numbness/disbelief (6 items) (Jacobs et al. 1986), 4) the short form (7 items) of the Texas Inventory of Grief (Faschingbauer et al. 1977), and 5) a self-rating of the severity of grief (scale of 0–4).

The subjects were then contacted to arrange a face-to-face interview. The interview was conducted by a psychiatrist and included a semistructured clinical interview, a structured assessment for pathologic grief, and questions about risk factors. The interview included the parts of the Structured Clinical Interview for DSM-III that assess major depression, panic disorder, and GAD. DSM-III-R hierarchical rules for diagnosis were not applied so that a participant could receive any or all of the diagnoses. Most of the participants were not assessed for anxiety disorders, as the original aim of the study was to examine only the relationship between pathologic grief and depressive syndromes. The assessment of anxiety disorders was completed on only 17 of the participants.

The structured assessment of pathologic grief was based on descriptive criteria developed specifically for the study. The conceptual framework of attachment theory provided the paradigm for the criteria. The diagnosis of pathologic grief was established by the clinical history or observation of the manifestations of separation distress.

The criteria defined four subtypes of pathologic grief: severe, delayed, prolonged, and absent. Specifically, the criteria required that the separation distress symptoms be of sufficient severity to receive a clinical rating of 4 on a scale of 1–4, or that the time course of separation distress symptoms be abnormal (i.e., delayed [onset 2 weeks or more after the loss] or prolonged [no change or worse 6 months after the loss]). Finally, the failure to report or observe any manifestations of separation distress constituted an absence of symptoms, a variant of pathologic grief. Although the assessment was structured, the psychiatric interviewer was not blind with respect to the diagnoses of major depression or anxiety disorder.

Results. The sample consisted of 25 bereaved spouses, the majority of whom were widows (92%). The average age was 51 years; 68% had completed high school, and 56% were employed.

Of the 25 participants, 16 (64%) met criteria for pathologic grief (see Table 7–3). With regard to the subtypes of pathologic grief, 1 participant (6%) met criteria for absent separation distress, 2 (12%) for delayed separation distress, 11 (69%) for severe separation distress, and 15 (94%) for prolonged separation distress. The subtypes of pathologic grief were not exclusive; 12 participants met criteria for one or more subtype. There were no significant differences in sociodemographic characteristics between those who met criteria for pathologic grief and those who did not.

The group with pathologic grief was significantly more likely to be diagnosed with major depression (94% versus 33%, $\chi^2 =$ 10.4, $P < .001$) than those without pathologic grief (see Table 7–3). The group with pathologic grief were more likely to be diagnosed with anxiety disorders (GAD: 82% versus 67%, panic disorder: 36% versus 17%) than those without pathologic grief, but these differences were not significant. When subtypes of pathologic grief were examined in relationship to depression and anxiety disorders, the two participants with the subtype of delayed separation distress were also diagnosed with major depressive episode 1 year after the loss of spouse. This was a confirmation of a relationship between delayed separation distress and major depression that was originally noted by Parkes (1972). Panic disorder was exclusively associated with the subtype of severe separation distress.

The group with pathologic grief scored significantly higher than those without pathologic grief on separation distress measures ($t = 3$, $P \leq .001$), PERI anxiety ($t = 2.9$, $P \leq .01$), and the CES-D ($t = 2.4$, $P \leq .05$). Those with pathologic grief also tended to score higher on self-rated grief, numbness/disbelief, and the Texas Inventory of Grief; these differences, however, were not statistically significant.

To summarize, pathologic grief was not isomorphic with depression, panic disorder, or GAD but did overlap with these disorders. Isomorphism was greatest for pathologic grief and major depression and least for pathologic grief and panic disorder. The group with pathologic grief scored significantly higher on the separation distress measures, the PERI anxiety scale, and the CES-D than the group without pathologic grief.

Risk Factors for Psychiatric Complications

In the study of risk factors, prospective studies are the most powerful designs because they provide baseline data on individuals before the bereavement. Among adults, the rate of bereavement for an immediate family member is only about 5% per year

Table 7–3. Cross-tabulations of bereaved persons with pathologic grief and those without pathologic grief by the presence or absence of panic disorder, generalized anxiety disorder (GAD), and major depressive disorder

| | Pathologic grief | | | | Total |
| | Present | | Absent | | |
Psychiatric disorder	n	%	n	%	n
Panic disorder present	4	36	1	17	5
Panic disorder absent	7	64	5	83	12
Total	11		6		17
GAD present	9	82	4	67	13
GAD absent	2	18	2	33	4
Total	11		6		17
Depression present	15	94*	3	33	18
Depression absent	1	6	6	67	7
Total	16		9		25

*$P \leq .001$.

(Osterweis et al. 1984), and the rate of psychiatric complications varies from 4% to 39% (Kim and Jacobs 1991). Therefore, an extremely large sample is necessary to determine whether a risk factor is associated with a particular psychiatric complication of bereavement. Most of the studies cited in this section are not prospective; they are comparisons of recently bereaved persons with control groups matched for relevant characteristics. In addition, the risk factors vary with the psychiatric complication. The risk factors are divided into three groups: personal factors, social factors, and factors associated with the death.

Personal factors.   During bereavement, women are at greater risk for depression and, to a lesser extent, for pathologic grief (Jacobs 1993). In general, women are at increased risk for depression (Regier et al. 1988), and this increased risk has been attributed at least in part to the stresses of child rearing and marriage (Merikangas et al. 1985; Weissman and Klerman 1977). With respect to bereavement, there may be differences in the nature of women's attachment and grief and their risk for role strain and financial hardship.

Younger persons are also at higher risk for depression. Environmental factors may play a role: trauma causes about 10% of the deaths per year in the United States, and it is the leading cause of death among persons under the age of 30. The frequency of traumatic loss may be the major reason for an increased risk of depression. For example, one study found that 40% of young adults were exposed to traumatic events, and 25% of those exposed developed PTSD (Breslau et al. 1991); 17% of the traumatic events were the sudden death or injury of family or friends.

There has been a great deal of research that examines the kinship to the deceased, and there are significant differences in the risk for complications. The odds of being depressed 4 months after a loss were significantly higher for a spouse than for children, siblings, or more distant relatives (McHorney and Mor 1988). The death of a spouse, parent, or child was significantly associated with depression within a year of the loss rather than the death of a sibling, grandchild, or good friend (Murrell and Himmelfarb 1989). In another study, Cleiren (1991) found that at 14 months, 15% of the spouses had severe depressive symptoms, and 31% of the parents were depressed.

Other researchers have focused on the nature of the survivor's attachment to the deceased. Freud (1917/1962) noted that ambivalent (and narcissistic) relationships place a person at greater risk for depression. However, ambivalence was not uniquely associated with narcissistic attachments and depressive reactions (Abraham 1924/1960; Siggens 1966). Freud's hypothesis has not been specifically tested in bereaved persons. Parkes and Weiss (1983) found that 38 bereaved spouses who reported high levels of marital conflict (two or more areas) had significantly worse outcomes 2 and 4 years after a loss as compared with spouses with low conflict. The high conflict group displayed a pattern of delayed grief. However, the conflict may have been related to illness in the family, to socioeconomic status, or both. Parkes and Weiss also found that dependent relationships were associated with chronic grief syndrome.

Some researchers question whether pathologic grief is a reflection of existing personality disorders (Alarcon 1984; Middleton et al. 1993). Bereavement may overwhelm an individual's ability to cope, upset a marginal state of adaptation, and exacerbate a preexisting personality disorder. Widowhood was associated with a diagnosis of borderline personality disorder in one epidemiologic survey (Swartz et al. 1990), but there were no baseline data on the respondents. In some cases, neurotic behaviors are a result of the psychiatric complications of bereavement. For example, episodes of depression can cause increases in introversion, dependency, neurosis, and emotional lability (Hirschfeld et al. 1989).

Bereaved persons with high scores on neuroticism and low sense of internal control were at high risk for depression, particularly with an unexpected loss (Raphael and Middleton 1990; Stroebe and Stroebe 1987). In contrast, there is no specific relationship between ego defenses and outcome. Widows with high scores on neurotic ego defenses 2 months after the death of a spouse were more likely to have high scores on depression scales 13 months after a loss (Jacobs et al. 1991; Kim et al. 1991).

It is not clear that positive personal and family histories of major depression are risk factors for depression in bereaved persons. Some studies fail to prove an association (Bruce et al. 1990;

Jacobs et al. 1989); others find that a past personal history of depression increases the risk twofold (Richards and McCallum 1979; Zisook and Shuchter 1991). In one study, a history of mental illness (major affective disorder, alcoholism, hysteria, undiagnosed illness) was a risk factor for depression. However, a history of major affective disorder was both rare and was not independently a risk factor in the same study (Bornstein et al. 1973). Jacobs et al. (1990) found that a past personal history of anxiety disorder or major depression and a family history of anxiety disorders were associated with a higher risk of panic disorder or GAD.

Childhood losses of a parent increased depressive risk by two- or threefold in one study (Lloyd 1980), although there is still debate over whether it is the actual loss or the consequences of the loss that is important. Tennant (1988) concluded that it was the failure to provide substitute nurturance in the circumstances of the loss that was associated with a later risk of major depression. Kendler et al. (1992) found that parental loss accounted for 1.5%–5.1% of the risk of developing depression later in life.

Social factors. In four longitudinal studies, there was little evidence that objective characteristics, such as number of close friends or number of contacts with others per week, have a long-term effect on adaptation to bereavement. In three of the studies, there was some evidence that the social environment affects emotional distress up to 2 months after the loss; after 2 months, the social network or support had no effect (Dimond et al. 1987; Hays 1991; Stroebe and Stroebe 1987).

In their study, Dimond et al. (1987) used a composite index of personal perception (subjective characteristics, such as closeness to network members and opportunity to express oneself) and objective characteristics of the social environment (number of contacts, frequency of confidences, amount of mutual help) to assess the social environment. Elderly persons with a positive composite index were less likely to be depressed at 2 months. This effect disappeared at later assessments (6–24 months). Objective characteristics, such as network size, strength, and density, had no relationship to depression at 2 months or later. In Stroebe and Stroebe's (1987) study, the size of the social network had no buffering effect on the depressive symptoms of bereavement for 2 years of follow-up. In a New Haven, Connecticut, study, only the density (number of persons in the network who knew each other) of the network was associated with outcome at 13 and 25 months after bereavement (Hays 1991).

In the fourth study, the only variable associated with persistent distress or unresolved grief was a perceived deficit in social supports measured 2 years after the loss (Vachon et al. 1982). Perceived deficits were not predictive of outcome but rather associated cross-sectionally with persistently high levels of emotional distress at 2 years (Vachon et al. 1982). Thus, the characteristics of the antecedent social environment did not predict bereavement outcome.

Two early, related studies also found that the bereaved person's perception of nonsupportiveness was associated with poor general health status scores 13 months after bereavement (Maddison and Viola 1968; Maddison and Walker 1967). Another study of bereaved persons whose partners or friends died of acquired immunodeficiency syndrome found that those who perceived that the emotional and instrumental support that they received was inadequate grieved more intensely than those with a positive perception of their support (Lennon et al. 1990). The availability of support was not related to the intensity of grief.

Is perceived nonsupportiveness related to the bereaved's personal view, or is it an actual deficiency of the social network? In one study, personality factors governed the state of loneliness of the neurotically depressed and anxious patients who were examined in the circumstances of stress (Henderson et al. 1981). In a prospective study, community-dwelling elderly with high depression scores reported having less emotionally satisfying and consistent support from relatives (Grant et al. 1988). These findings indicate that the individual's anxious, depressed state rather than the social network determines the perception of nonsupport. These studies suggest that perceived nonsupportiveness is more related to the bereaved's personal view than the social network.

Factors associated with the death. Untimely, unanticipated deaths from acute illness or trauma are associated with a higher risk of complications during bereavement. There is one exception. Among the elderly, chronic illnesses before a death are associated with more difficult bereavement (Heyman and Gianturco 1973; Sanders 1989).

As noted, trauma causes about 10% of deaths per year in the United States. Survivors of traumatic or unnatural events respond with horror and fears of vulnerability, and they view the environment as desolate and dangerous (van der Kolk and van der Hart 1989). Death evokes self-protective reactions: denial, dissociation of the reality from consciousness, avoidance, and a failure to integrate the death cognitively (Horowitz 1986). In addition, traumatic bereavement has a higher risk for major depression, anxiety disorder, and PTSD (Shore et al. 1986) than nontraumatic bereavement, with some exceptions (Cleiren 1991; Lundin 1984). There is preliminary evidence that traumatic losses can induce "traumatic distress," a distinct dimension of grief. For example, schoolchildren exposed to a terrorist shooting experienced both separation distress and traumatic distress (fear, horror, vulnerability, disintegration of cognitive assumptions) secondary to the death of their schoolmates (Nader et al. 1990; Pynoos et al. 1987). Moreover, life events researchers argue that the specific qualities of experiences have a relationship to particular qualities of the subsequent emotional distress (Finlay-Jones and Brown 1981). Thus, fear-provoking life events lead to higher risk for anxiety disorders, and loss-related life events lead to higher risk for depressive disorders.

Traumatic distress symptoms occur frequently. In a study of 128 bereaved adults whose family members had died of multiple causes, 60%–80% of the sample experienced intrusive and avoidant traumatic symptoms (Schut et al. 1991). The symptoms occurred over 25 months of bereavement, with 20%–31% of participants meeting criteria for PTSD at some point of the study, and 9% meeting criteria throughout the course of the study. Cardiac and cancer deaths were the primary causes of the deaths that caused the traumatic distress symptoms. The traumatic symptomatology was associated with not having anticipated the loss and not having taken leave of the person. Unnatural and traumatic causes of death were rare and not associated with PTSD.

Summary. Different risk factors exist for major depression, anxiety disorders, and pathologic grief. Women and younger persons are at higher risk for major depression. Those with a history of depression or anxiety and a family history of anxiety are at higher risk for anxiety disorders. Social networks decrease emotional distress in the first 2 months of bereavement, but the effect disappears after 2 months. Traumatic deaths are associated with depression, GAD, and PTSD. Unanticipated deaths are associated with PTSD and pathologic grief. Given the absence of prospective studies, these findings should be viewed as preliminary.

CLINICAL IMPLICATIONS OF COMPLICATED BEREAVEMENT

In this last section, we discuss the use of psychotherapeutic and psychotropic methods to treat the psychiatric complications of bereavement. There have been no randomized clinical trials of psychotherapeutic or psychotropic interventions in bereavement. We have chosen several psychotherapeutic interventions that have been developed based on small clinical trials or that represent current cognitive approaches. We also present information based on open trials of psychotropic medications or clinical observations of efficacy.

Psychotherapeutic Interventions

The clinician should begin psychotherapeutic treatment with a thorough evaluation, including a detailed history of the death, the bereaved's immediate and subsequent reactions to the loss, a review of previous losses, and an evaluation of ways of coping with past problems (Raphael 1975, 1983). The duration of treatment should be brief, 10–15 meetings. The clinician should be explicit about the duration of treatment from the beginning. Either a brief psychodynamic approach (Horowitz et al. 1984) or a brief confrontational and behavioral approach (Mawson et al. 1981) is effective most of the time. At the end of treatment, the clinician should review the process of treatment and explore the patient's feelings about its conclusion.

Parkes and Weiss (1983) identified specific types of psycho-therapy for different types of pathologic grief. For patients who present with sudden, unexpected grief syndromes, they recommended supportive and pacing strategies to address the overwhelming reality of the loss and the accompanying feelings. For patients who present with ambivalent feelings and delayed grief, they recommended using confrontational or counterphobic strategies to address the avoidance of grief. For patients with a dependent relationship to the deceased and prolonged grief, they recommended using a supportive and goal-oriented approach with an insistence on the patient's development of autonomy. Rynearson (1987) wrote about patients with traumatic losses and recommended focusing on the sense of desolation as well as the consequences of the trauma: victimization and fear of recurrent violence.

For patients with different character styles, Horowitz et al. (1984) identified particular "target" issues. Patients with obsessional styles may use intellectual explanations to enhance their sense of control, but clinicians should encourage them to explore the emotional aspects of the experience. Patients with hysterical styles may express emotional aspects easily, but clinicians may have to reinforce the need for interpretation of the meaning and conceptual implications of the loss. Each patient will interact with the therapist in a way that reflects the self-images and role relationships that govern his or her behavior with intimates and authority figures (Horowitz et al. 1980, 1984). The clinician can learn about past attachments, unresolved issues with the deceased, and past losses, and incorporate this information into the treatment.

Jacobs (1993) has advocated psychoeducation as a cornerstone of psychotherapy for the bereaved. The psychoeducational approach is integrated with a psychodynamically sophisticated appreciation of the person's adaptation to the loss, is attentive to interpersonal problems, and uses cognitive-behavioral interventions as specific strategies during the course of bereavement. The clinician encourages the patient to do the emotional tasks of experiencing the pain of the loss, the cognitive tasks of changing one's assumptions about the world secondary to the loss, and social tasks such as developing new skills and role models (Raphael 1975; Shuchter 1986; Worden 1982). Jacobs (1993) stresses the importance of educating the patient about bereavement and providing reasonable expectations based on current knowledge of bereavement (e.g., normalize angry feelings about being left behind).

Psychotropic Interventions

Treatment of anxiety disorders. Most researchers and clinicians agree with the use of anxiolytics and hypnotics briefly in the first few days of unexpected bereavement (Hollister 1972; Osterweis et al. 1984). In general, benzodiazepines are indicated as brief treatment for anxiety disorders such as panic and disabling GAD (Rickels and Schweitzer 1987). Target symptoms are panic attacks and anticipatory anxiety. Since GAD occurs seldomly without panic disorder (Kim and Jacobs 1991), GAD is not a useful indication for treatment.

Benzodiazepines are also useful in treating the emotional and autonomic arousal, severe anxiety, and intrusive symptoms of PTSD (Forster and Marmar 1991). Preclinical evidence indicates that benzodiazepines reduce the dysregulation in neurophysiologic function caused by severe stress and that they can prevent the maladaptive behavioral states associated with experimentally induced traumatic disorders (Bremner et al. 1991; Forster and Marmar 1991). The preclinical data suggest the potential to avert the development of PTSD. Target symptoms are intrusive images, nightmares, startle reactions, hypervigilance, tremor, tachycardia, palpitations, sweating, and difficulty falling or staying asleep. Avoidant symptoms, such as emotional numbing, emotional constriction, and feeling stunned or dazed, are less likely to improve with benzodiazepines.

Before prescribing benzodiazepines, the clinician should consider certain issues. A history of alcohol abuse and a histrionic character style may be associated with a higher risk of disinhibition of behavior with benzodiazepines (Forster and Marmar 1991). Benzodiazepines can interfere with cognitive and memory functions and should be used with caution in circumstances of sudden or traumatic death because of possible amnestic reactions (Tyrer 1983). There are mixed reports as to whether the bereaved are at greater risk for developing dependence (Forster and Marmar 1991; Tyrer 1983; Zisook et al. 1990). Some researchers believe that anxiolytics have the potential for causing "frozen" grief (Hamlin and Hammersley 1988; Rynearson et al. 1990). They hypothesized that benzodiazepines interfere with cognitive processing of the loss or promote a greater use of denial and avoidance as coping strategies. Nevertheless, there is no good evidence as yet that the supervised use of anxiolytics interferes with the resolution of grief in carefully screened patients (Jacobs 1993).

Treatment of major depression. Preclinical data indicate that imipramine has been effective in reversing the depressive behavior and social withdrawal of primates separated from their mothers or siblings. Imipramine has also prevented the emergence of depressive behaviors in highly aroused primates exposed to the stress of loss (McKinney 1985). In a small, uncontrolled clinical trial of desipramine, there was a positive response with improved sleep within 1 week and improvement in other symptoms in 2 weeks (Jacobs et al. 1987). An open trial of nortriptyline (Pasternak et al. 1991) was also positive. The target symptoms for antidepressants are dysphoria, depressive cognition, and neurovegetative symptoms.

Before prescribing antidepressants, the clinician should consider certain issues. In the initial phase of treatment, tricyclics can precipitate or aggravate panic attacks. The clinician should distinguish between separation distress symptoms and depressive symptoms to avoid unnecessary increases in the dose of antidepressants.

Treatment of pathologic grief. There have been no systematic studies that examine the psychotropic interventions for pathologic grief. Anecdotal reports of the treatment of separation distress in adults include the use of doxepin in one case and amitriptyline in another (Shuchter 1982). However, desipramine did not decrease separation distress in a small study (Jacobs et al. 1987).

Treatment of psychotic symptoms. Jacobs (1993) cautioned against inappropriate use of antipsychotic medications, as psychotic decompensation is uncommon in bereavement. However, illusions and hallucinations associated with the deceased do occur. In one study, 47% of conjugally bereaved individuals experienced illusions (feeling the presence of the deceased) or hallucinations (14% had visual hallucinations, 13% had auditory hallucinations) (Rees 1971). The visually impaired elderly may experience visual hallucinations that are more related to sensory deprivation (Adair and Keshavan 1988; Alroe and McIntyre 1983) and do not require antipsychotics.

CONCLUSION

Bereavement is a severe stressor that increases an individual's risk for psychiatric disorders. The rate ranges of psychiatric complications are 4%–34% for pathologic grief, 17%–31% for major depression, and 13%–39% for anxiety disorders. Unanticipated deaths are associated with a higher risk for pathologic grief and PTSD; traumatic deaths are associated with a higher risk for major depression, GAD, and PTSD. Women and younger persons are at higher risk for major depression complicating bereavement. Although there are no controlled clinical trials of treatment of the psychiatric complications of bereavement, there is some evidence that both psychotherapeutic and psychotropic interventions may be effective.

REFERENCES

Abraham K: A short study of the development of the libido, viewed in the light of mental disorders (1924), in Selected Papers on Psychoanalysis. Translated by Bryan D, Strachey A. New York, Basic Books, 1960, pp 418–501

Adair DK, Keshavan MS: The Charles Bonnet syndrome and grief reaction (letter). Am J Psychiatry 145:895–896, 1988

Adler A: Neuropsychiatric complications in victims of Boston's Coconut Grove disaster. JAMA 123:1098–1101, 1943

Alarcon RD: Personality disorder as a pathogenic factor in bereavement. J Nerv Ment Dis 172:45–47, 1984

Alroe CJ, McIntyre JNM: Visual hallucinations: the Charles Bonnet syndrome and bereavement. Med J Aust 2:674–675, 1983

American Psychiatric Association: Diagnostic and Statistical Manual of Mental Disorders, 3rd Edition, Revised. Washington, DC, American Psychiatric Association, 1987

Barrett CJ, Schneweis KM: An empirical search for stages of widowhood. Omega 11:97–105, 1980

Birtchnell J: The relationship between attempted suicide, depression, and parent death. Br J Psychiatry 116:307–313, 1970

Blanchard CG, Blanchard EB, Becker JV: The young widow: depressive symptomatology through the grief process. Psychiatry 39:394–399, 1976

Bornstein PE, Clayton PJ, Halikas JA, et al: The depression of widowhood after thirteen months. Br J Psychiatry 122:561–566, 1973

Bowlby J: Attachment and Loss, Vol 2: Separation. New York, Basic Books, 1973

Bowlby J: Attachment and Loss, Vol 3: Loss, Sadness and Depression. New York, Basic Books, 1980

Bowlby J, Parkes CM: Separation and loss, in The International Yearbook for Child Psychiatry and Allied Disciplines, Vol 1: The Child and His Family. New York, Wiley, 1970, pp 197–216

Bremner JD, Southwick SM, Charney DS: Animal models for the neurobiology of trauma. Posttraumatic Stress Disorder Research Quarterly 2:1–7, 1991

Breslau N, Davis GC, Andreski P, et al: Traumatic events and posttraumatic stress disorder in an urban population of young adults. Arch Gen Psychiatry 48:216–222, 1991

Bruce ML, Kim K, Leaf PJ, et al: Depressive episodes and dysphoria resulting from conjugal bereavement in a prospective community sample. Am J Psychiatry 147:608–611, 1990

Clayton PJ, Darvish HS: Course of depressive symptoms following the stress of bereavement, in Stress and Mental Disorder. Edited by Barrett JE, Rose RM, Klerman GL, et al. New York, Raven, 1979, pp 121–136

Clayton PJ, Halikas JA, Maurice WL: The bereavement of the widowed. Diseases of the Nervous System 32:597–604, 1971

Clayton PJ, Herjanic M, Murphy GE, et al: Mourning and depression: their similarities and differences. Canadian Psychiatric Association Journal 19:309–313, 1974

Cleiren MPHD: Adaptation After Bereavement. Leiden, The Netherlands, DSWO Press, 1991

Comstock GW, Helsing KJ: Symptoms of depression in two communities. Psychol Med 6:551–563, 1976

Darwin C: The Expression of the Emotions in Man and Animals. London, John Murray, 1872

Deutsch H: Absence of grief. Psychoanal Q 6:12–22, 1937

Dimond M, Lund DA, Caserta MS: The role of social support in the first two years of bereavement in an elderly sample. Gerontologist 27:599–604, 1987

Dohrenwend BP, Shrout PE, Egri G, et al: Nonspecific psychological distress and other dimensions of psychopathology. Arch Gen Psychiatry 37:1229–1236, 1980

Elliott GR, Eisdorfer C (eds): Stress and Human Health: A Study by the Institute of Medicine, National Academy of Sciences. New York, Springer, 1982

Engel G: Sudden and rapid death during psychological stress. Ann Intern Med 74:771–782, 1971

Faschingbauer TR, DeVaul R, Zisook S: Development of the Texas Inventory of Grief. Am J Psychiatry 134:696–698, 1977

Finlay-Jones R, Brown G: Types of stressful life event and the onset of anxiety and depressive disorders. Psychol Med 11:803–815, 1981

Forster P, Marmar CR: Benzodiazepines in acute stress reactions: benefits, risks, and controversies, in Benzodiazepines in Clinical Practice: Risks and Benefits. Edited by Roy-Byrne PP, Cowley DS. Washington, DC, American Psychiatric Press, 1991, pp 73–89

Freud S: Mourning and melancholia (1917), in The Standard Edition of the Complete Psychological Works of Sigmund Freud, Vol 14. Translated and edited by Strachey J. London, Hogarth Press, 1962, pp 243–258

Grant I, Patterson TL, Yager J: Social supports in relation to physical health and symptoms of depression in the elderly. Am J Psychiatry 145:1254–1258, 1988

Hamlin M, Hammersley D: Benzodiazepines following bereavement. Paper presented at the International Conference on Grief and Bereavement in Contemporary Society, London, July 1988

Hays JC: Psychological distress, social environment, and seeking social support following conjugal bereavement. Unpublished doctoral dissertation, Yale University School of Epidemiology and Public Health, New Haven, CT, 1991

Helsing KJ, Szklo M, Comstock GW: Factors associated with mortality after widowhood. Am J Public Health 71:802–809, 1981

Helsing KJ, Comstock GW, Szklo M: Causes of death in a widowed population. Am J Epidemiol 116:524–532, 1982

Henderson S, Byrne DG, Duncan-Jones P: Neurosis and the Social Environment. New York, Academic Press, 1981

Heyman DK, Gianturco DT: Long term adaptation by the elderly to bereavement. J Gerontol 28:259–262, 1973

Hirschfeld RMA, Klerman GL, Lavori P, et al: Premorbid personality assessments of first onset of major depression. Arch Gen Psychiatry 46:345–350, 1989

Hollister L: Psychotherapeutic drugs in the dying and bereaved. Journal of Thanatology 2:623–629, 1972

Holmes RH, Rahe RH: The social readjustment rating scale. J Psychosom Res 11:213–218, 1967

Horowitz MJ: Stress Response Syndromes. New York, Jason Aronson, 1976

Horowitz MJ: Stress response syndromes: a review of posttraumatic and adjustment disorders. Hosp Community Psychiatry 37:241–249, 1986

Horowitz MJ, Wilner N, Alvarez W: Impact of Event Scale: a measure of subjective stress. Psychosom Med 41:209–218, 1979

Horowitz MJ, Wilner N, Marmar C, et al: Pathological grief and the activation of latent self-images. Am J Psychiatry 137:1157–1162, 1980

Horowitz MJ, Marmar C, Krupnick J, et al: Personality Styles and Brief Psychotherapy. New York, Basic Books, 1984

Jacobs SC: Bereavement and anxiety disorders, in Grief and Bereavement in Contemporary Society, Vol 1. Edited by Chigier E. London, Freund Publishing, 1987, pp 212–220

Jacobs SC: Pathologic Grief: Maladaptation to Loss. Washington, DC, American Psychiatric Press, 1993

Jacobs SC, Kim K: Psychiatric complications of bereavement. Psychiatric Annals 20:314–317 1990

Jacobs SC, Kasl SV, Ostfeld AM, et al: The measurement of grief: bereaved versus non-bereaved. Hospice Journal 2:21–36, 1986

Jacobs SC, Nelson JC, Zisook S: Treating depressions of bereavement with antidepressants: a pilot study. Psychiatr Clin North Am 10:501–510, 1987

Jacobs SC, Hansen FF, Berkman L, et al: Depressions of bereavement. Compr Psychiatry 30:218–224, 1989

Jacobs SC, Hansen FF, Kasl SV, et al: Anxiety disorders during acute bereavement: risk and risk factors. J Clin Psychiatry 51:269–274, 1990

Jacobs SC, Kim K, Schaefer C, et al: Coping styles, ego defenses, and outcome following bereavement. Paper presented at the Third International Conference on Grief and Bereavement, Sydney, Australia, June 1991

Kendler KS, Neale MC, Kessler RC, et al: Childhood parental loss and adult psychopathology in women. Arch Gen Psychiatry 49:109–116, 1992

Kim K, Jacobs SC: Pathologic grief and its relationship to other psychiatric disorders. J Affect Disord 21:257–263, 1991

Kim K, Jacobs S, Schaefer C, et al: Conscious and unconscious coping under stress; I: relationship to each other and neuroendocrine function. Paper presented at the Third International Conference on Grief and Bereavement, Sydney, Australia, June 1991

Lennon MC, Martin JL, Dean L: The influence of social support on AIDS-related grief reaction among gay men. Soc Sci Med 31:477–484, 1990

Lindemann EL: Symptomatology and management of acute grief. Am J Psychiatry 101:141–148, 1944

Lloyd C: Live events and depressive disorders reviewed. Arch Gen Psychiatry 37:529–535, 1980

Lundin T: Long-term outcome of bereavement. Br J Psychiatry 145:414–428, 1984

MacMahon B, Pugh RF: Suicide in the widowed. Am J Epidemiol 81:23–31, 1965

Maddison D, Viola A: The health of widows in the year following bereavement. J Psychosom Res 12:297–306, 1968

Maddison DC, Walker WL: Factors affecting the outcome of conjugal bereavement. Br J Psychiatry 113:1057–1068, 1967

Mawson D, Marks IM, Ramm L, et al: Guided mourning for morbid grief: a controlled study. Br J Psychiatry 138:185–193, 1981

McHorney CA, Mor V: Predictors of bereavement depression and its health services consequences. Med Care 26:882–893, 1988

McKinney WT: Separation and depression: biological markers, in The Psychobiology of Attachment and Separation. Edited by Reite M, Field T. New York, Academic Press, 1985, pp 201–222

Merikangas KR, Weissman MM, Pauls DL: Genetic factors in the sex ratio of major depression. Psychol Med 15:63–69, 1985

Middleton W, Raphael B, Martinek N, et al: Pathologic grief reactions, in Handbook of Bereavement: Theory, Research, and Intervention. Edited by Strocbe MS, Strocbe W, Hansson RO. Cambridge, Cambridge Univerity Press, 1993, pp 44–61

Murphy GE, Armstrong MD, Heremele SL, et al: Suicide and alcoholism. Arch Gen Psychiatry 36:65–69, 1979

Murrell SA, Himmelfarb S: Effects of attachment bereavement and pre-event conditions on subsequent depressive symptoms in older adults. Psychol Aging 4:166–172, 1989

Nader K, Pynoos RS, Fairbanks L, et al: Childhood PTSD reactions one year after a sniper attack. Am J Psychiatry 147:1526–1530, 1990

Osterweis M, Solomon F, Green M (eds): Bereavement: Reactions, Consequences and Care. Washington, DC, National Academy Press, 1984

Parkes CM: Bereavement: Studies of Grief in Adult Life. New York, International Universities Press, 1972

Parkes CM, Weiss RS: Recovery From Bereavement. New York, Basic Books, 1983

Pasternak RE, Reynolds CF, Schlernitzauer M, et al: Acute open-trial nortriptyline therapy of bereavement-related depression in late life. J Clin Psychiatry 52:307–310, 1991

Pynoos RS, Frederick C, Nader K, et al: Life threat and posttraumatic stress in school-age children. Arch Gen Psychiatry 44:1057–1063, 1987

Raphael B: The management of pathological grief. Aust N Z J Psychiatry 9:173–180, 1975

Raphael B: The Anatomy of Bereavement. New York, Basic Books, 1983

Raphael B, Middleton W: Pathologic bereavement: what is pathologic grief? Psychiatric Annals 20:304–307, 1990

Rees WD: The hallucinations of widowhood. BMJ 4:37–41, 1971

Rees WD, Lutkins SG: Mortality of bereavement. BMJ 4:13–16, 1967

Regier DA, Boyd JH, Burke JD, et al: One month prevalence of mental disorders in the United States. Arch Gen Psychiatry 45:977–988, 1988

Richards JG, McCallum J: Bereavement in the elderly. N Z Med J 89:201–204, 1979

Rickels K, Schweitzer EE: Current pharmacotherapy of anxiety and panic, in Psychopharmacology: The Third Generation of Progress. Edited by Meltzer HY. New York, Raven, 1987, pp 1193–1203

Rynearson EK, Jacobs SC, Marmar CR: Pathologic grief. Psychiatric Update 10:1–9, 1990

Rynearson EK: Psychological adjustment to unnatural dying, in Biopsychosocial Aspects of Bereavement. Edited by Zisook S. Washington, DC, American Psychiatric Press, 1987, pp 75–93

Sanders CM: Grief: The Mourning After. New York, Wiley, 1989

Schut HAW, de Keijser J, van den Bout J: Incidence and prevalence of post-traumatic symptomatology in conjugally bereaved. Abstract presented at the Third International Conference on Grief and Bereavement in Contemporary Society. Sydney, Australia, June 1991

Shore JM, Tatum EL, Vollmer WM: Psychiatric reactions to disaster. Am J Psychiatry 143:590–595, 1986

Shuchter SR: The depression of widowhood reconsidered: the role of antidepressants. Paper presented at the annual meeting of the American Psychiatric Association, Toronto, Ontario, Canada, May 1982

Shuchter SR: Dimensions of Grief: Adjusting to the Death of a Spouse. San Francisco, CA, Jossey-Bass, 1986

Siggens LD: Mourning: a critical survey of the literature. Int J Psychoanal 47:14–25, 1966

Silverman P: Widow to Widow. New York, Springer, 1986

Spitzer RL, Williams BW, Gibbon M: Structured Clinical Interview for DSM-III. New York, Biometrics Research, 1985

Stein Z, Susser M: Widowhood and mental illness. British Journal of Preventive and Social Medicine 23:106–110, 1969

Stroebe W, Stroebe MS: Bereavement and Health. New York, Cambridge University Press, 1987

Swartz M, Blazer D, George L, et al: Estimating the prevalence of borderline personality disorder in the community. Journal of Personality Disorders 4:257–272, 1990

Tennant C: Parental loss in childhood. Arch Gen Psychiatry 45:1045–1050, 1988

Tyrer P: The place of tranquilizers in the management of stress. J Psychosom Res 27:385–389, 1983

Vachon MLS, Sheldon AR, Lancee WJ, et al: Correlates of enduring distress patterns following bereavement: social network, life situation, and personality. Psychol Med 12:783–788, 1982

van der Kolk BA, van der Hart O: Pierre Janet and the breakdown of adaptation in psychological trauma. Am J Psychiatry 146:1530–1540, 1989

Weissman MM, Klerman GL: Sex differences and the epidemiology of depression. Arch Gen Psychiatry 34:98–111, 1977

Weissman M, Sholomskas D, Pottenger M, et al: Assessing depressive symptoms in five psychiatric populations: a validation study. Am J Epidemiol 106:203–213, 1979

Windholz MJ, Marmar CR, Horowitz MJ: A review of the research on conjugal bereavement: impact on health and efficacy of intervention. Compr Psychiatry 26:433–437, 1985

Worden JW: Grief Counseling and Grief Therapy: A Handbook for the Mental Health Practitioner. New York, Springer, 1982

Wortman CB, Silver RC: The myths of coping with loss. J Consult Clin Psychol 57:349–357, 1989

Zisook S, DeVaul R: Grief, unresolved grief, and depression. Psychosomatics 24:247–256, 1983

Zisook S, Shuchter SR: Depression through the first year after the death of a spouse. Am J Psychiatry 148:1346–1352, 1991

Zisook S, Schneider D, Schuchter SR: Anxiety and bereavement. Psychol Med 8:83–96, 1990

Chapter 8

Preventive Interventions in the Workplace to Reduce Negative Psychiatric Consequences of Work and Family Stress

David L. Snow, Ph.D., and Marsha L. Kline, Ph.D.

P reventive interventions in the workplace involve strategies to reduce the onset of psychiatric disorders. The focus of these strategies is to modify known risk factors (e.g., work and family stressors) or to promote competencies as protection against dysfunction. They also involve efforts characterized by early identification and intervention with individuals exhibiting initial signs of problem formation, who are therefore at particularly high risk of developing a disorder.

The design and implementation of these types of interventions require a framework for guiding the process of knowledge development and utilization. One useful schema for the prevention research process (Price 1983) involves four interrelated domains. Initially, once a problem area has been defined, models are formulated to guide basic, descriptive studies of the problem. The knowledge derived from these studies then aids in the identification of modifiable risk and protective factors, which in turn inform the development of preventive interventions. Intervention methodologies are selected and introduced and then evaluated and refined until they can be disseminated systematically, with

This research was supported in part by a grant from the National Institute on Drug Abuse (R01 DA05205), David L. Snow, principal investigator, and Marsha L. Kline, co-investigator.

the expected outcome of reduction in the incidence and prevalence of the disorder. The extent to which these outcomes have
been achieved then can be tested, leading to reformulation of the
initial problem definition and the beginning of the cycle over
again.

This schema has direct relevance to research on work and
family stress. The defined problem area in this case involves
questions about how work and family stressors contribute to
negative psychiatric consequences. A clear rationale exists for
studying such relationships within the context of the workplace
and family. The workplace represents a critical social setting due
to its centrality and pervasive influence in the lives of adults. It is,
therefore, an excellent laboratory for conducting stress-related
research. It provides access to a substantial portion of the adult
population, ranging from those at risk but asymptomatic to those
showing early signs of symptomatology to those in need of treatment. In addition, there is a need to determine the extent to
which the workplace has an impact in positive and negative
ways on adult development and adjustment.

However, processes within the workplace account for only a
portion of the variance in individual adjustment, since factors in
nonwork contexts also contribute to these outcomes. The nonwork context of comparable centrality for adults is the family.
The boundary between work and family domains is increasingly
permeable; work stressors may be compounded by stressful life
events and conditions within the family and vice versa (e.g.,
Neale et al. 1983). Similarly, positive events or conditions in one
domain may serve to buffer negative circumstances within the
other domain. Thus, researchers need to identify risk and protective processes within and between these domains to identify
subgroups at greatest risk for mental health problems, substance
use problems, or both.

RESEARCH MODELS FOR STUDYING
THE STRESS PROCESS

Several models of the stress process are applicable to the development of research aimed at identifying crucial work and family

risk and protective factors and to the development of workplace preventive interventions. Theories about the nature of this process provide explanatory models for studying the relationship between stressors (either chronic conditions or significant life events) and negative health outcomes, including psychiatric symptomatology. A transactional model, proposed by Lazarus and Folkman (1984), places emphasis on the interaction between person and environment. This model has been instrumental in explaining how an individual may be more or less vulnerable to given sources of stress. According to this view, stress processes occur within important situational contexts rather than in isolation. Thus, it is assumed that relationships among stressors, coping processes, social support, and psychiatric disorders vary across settings and population subgroups.

A model posited by Moos and Swindle (1990) has five components, representing 1) the environmental system (stressors and social resources), 2) the personal system (demographics and personal factors), 3) life crisis or transition (event-related factors), 4) cognitive appraisal and coping responses, and 5) health and well-being outcomes. The model has been used to identify relationships between stressors and depression and between stressors and alcoholism.

Pearlin and Schooler (1978) addressed levels of individual change through a model that emphasizes coping as the primary concept. They defined a hierarchy of responses in which individuals can attempt to change a situation, control the meaning of a stressful event or experience, or manage the stress when it cannot be minimized or removed at its source. This model suggests strategies for enhancing individual coping by helping people to identify what options they have in a situation and to apply cognitive and social skills effectively based on these options.

Two organization-focused models also serve as relevant examples of theory development in this area of research. Kahn and Byosiere (1990) presented a structural view of the construct of work stress. In their model, they included organizational antecedents to stress; stressors in organizational life, such as role stressors; perceptions and cognitions (the appraisal process); and responses to stress, including psychiatric symptomatology. The linkages between these components of the model are mediated by properties of the person (e.g., self-esteem and locus of control) and properties of the situation (e.g., supervisor and coworker social support), with the ramifying consequences of stress assessed in terms of health and illness and organizational effectiveness.

A second work-related model, articulated by Ivancevich et al. (1990), is posed within an intervention framework. It explicates situational stressors, cognitive appraisals, and coping strategies as desired targets for interventions, regardless of whether the interventions attempt to influence the individual, the organization, or the individual-organizational interface. The desired outcomes of interventions again may be individual, organizational, or both, in nature.

Central to each of these models is the role of risk and protective factors in relation to psychiatric outcomes. Research aimed at identifying factors that exacerbate or mitigate psychopathology, as one of the early steps in the prevention research cycle, provides the empirical evidence for selecting relevant intervention strategies. Based on this knowledge, interventions are designed to reduce stressors, modify employees' perceptions, improve individuals' coping skills, and/or enhance social support (Heaney and van Ryn 1990; Ivancevich et al. 1990). In this way, the models provide a bridge between risk and protective factor research and intervention research.

Our purpose in this chapter is to review risk and protective factor and intervention research in the area of work and family stress, and then to present in detail empirical data regarding the effectiveness of a workplace coping-skills intervention conducted by the authors. First, we review evidence linking work and family stressors to psychiatric symptomatology. Second, we examine the role of social support from work and family sources and of individual coping strategies as protective factors in relation to psychiatric outcomes. Third, we summarize findings from previous studies regarding the effectiveness of workplace interventions in reducing negative psychiatric consequences. Fourth, we present a workplace intervention study—drawn from the Yale Work and Family Stress Project (Snow and Kline 1991a)—to illustrate issues regarding the design, implementation, and evaluation of preventive intervention strategies. Finally, we discuss implications for theory and future research pertaining to work and family stress.

WORK AND FAMILY STRESSORS: RELATIONSHIP TO PSYCHIATRIC OUTCOMES

The relationship between work and family stressors and psychiatric outcomes, including substance use, has been studied across a wide range of work settings, occupational groups, and demographic categories. Although much of the early research in this area focused primarily on the impact of various job stressors on men, in more recent years, with the increasing number of women entering the work force, investigations have begun to examine the influence of these types of stressors on both women and men. In addition, models to guide this research have been expanded to include stressors from family as well as work domains, acknowledging that individuals occupy multiple roles (e.g., worker, spouse, parent), each with its unique and overlapping sources of stress. Multiple-role occupancy increases the chances of experiencing higher levels of demand and of being exposed to a broader range of stressful conditions, as well as the potential for conflict between work and family domains. Whether these circumstances increase the likelihood of adverse health outcomes, or result in beneficial effects, has been the focus of increasing research interest. We first summarize empirical evidence regarding the impact of job-related stressors on psychiatric symptomatology and substance use and then review findings from studies examining work-family conflict and role strain.

Job or occupational stressors typically include measures of work load, responsibility pressure, role conflict, role ambiguity, and conflict with supervisors and coworkers. In general, job-related stressors correspond with a variety of negative outcomes for individuals across occupations, and stressful job settings have been associated with poor job performance, absenteeism, turnover, and burnout (Ivancevich and Matteson 1980). Job pressures and tensions operate as significant risk factors for health behavior (House et al. 1986), and poor interpersonal relationships at work have been tied to high levels of distress and anxiety (French and Caplan 1973; Kahn and Wolfe 1964).

A number of studies have involved blue-collar workers or other employee groups within industrial settings. In a 1-year longitudinal study of married, male, power-plant employees (Bromet et al. 1988), high levels of perceived work load, after controlling for age, were associated with an increase in symptoms of psychological distress, as well as increased risk of affective disorder. Perceived occupational stress was positively associated with disorders traditionally considered psychological and psychosomatic in another study of male, blue-collar workers (House et al. 1979). Similarly, in a sample of industrial supervisors, organizational role stress was positively related to neuroticism (Srivastava and Singh 1988). Two studies of factory workers, one conducted in Finland with male and female workers (Aro and Hasan 1987) and the other in Nigeria with male workers (Shankar and Famuyiwa 1991), add further corroborating evidence. In the Finnish study, psychosocial stressors at work were strongly associated with mental strain in men and women; in the Nigerian study, job stress had a negative impact on mental health, with increasing job pressure associated with deterioration in mental health status. Boxer and Wild (1992) found levels of psychological distress and alcohol problems to be higher than expected among fire fighters compared with typical community or working populations. The most striking finding was the increased likelihood of depression in workers reporting stressful relationships with supervisors. In a related study of primarily male police and fire department personnel (Fusilier et al. 1987), role ambiguity was positively related to depression. These studies of blue-collar and related occupational groups provide substantial evidence linking a range of job-related stressors to higher levels of psychiatric symptomatology.

Studies of individuals in professional and white-collar occupations provide further evidence supporting the relationship between work stressors and psychiatric symptoms. Among personnel from the teaching profession, job strain was related to depression and psychophysiologic symptoms (Schonfeld 1990); work stressors, particularly work load, were associated with increased frustration and anger, fatigue and health problems, and symptoms of burnout (Ratsoy et al. 1986). For one mixed sample of female and male clerical and management personnel (Hendrix et al. 1988), job stress correlated positively with burnout, defined as a syndrome of emotional exhaustion and cynicism toward one's work as a response to chronic stressors. In a large-scale study of white-collar workers in Sweden (Karasek et al. 1987), self-reported demands at work were associated with depressive symptomatology.

Investigations of other potentially high-stress occupational groups have included nursing personnel and mental health workers. Cooper and Baglioni (1988), using structural modeling in a study of nurse managers in England, found that personality and coping strategies preceded and determined the perception of job stressors, but the perception of job stressors then directly influenced mental well-being. Job stress was among the predictors of emotional exhaustion (feelings of depression, helplessness, hopelessness, and entrapment) for nurses in a neonatal intensive care unit (Oehler et al. 1991), and level of perceived job demand was associated with symptoms of depression in a sample of mostly female hospital and nursing home employees (Landsbergis 1988). Finally, higher scores on situational sources of organizational stress were positively related to a measure of total mood disturbance (with differences on tension-anxiety, depression-dejection, and confusion subscales) in male and female mental health direct care workers (Donat et al. 1991).

Evidence concerning the relationship between work stressors and substance use is less consistent than that reported for other types of psychiatric symptomatology. Harris and Fennell (1988) suggested that job stress may indirectly increase alcohol consumption by making drinking seem more useful for relieving stress, particularly if alcohol use is a part of the occupational culture. Job-related distress is associated with women's problem drinking only when particular adverse work experiences afflict women with particular personal characteristics and social circumstances. When these narrower implications of job stress are taken into account, work-related stressors explain only a small portion of the variance of problem drinking (Wilsnack and Wilsnack 1992).

Much of what influences employees' drinking may be due to factors outside the workplace. Hollinger (1988) investigated male and female employees most likely to work under the influence of alcohol or other drugs, reporting findings in support of Parker and Brody's (1982) contention that the phenomenon of working under the influence requires a multiple-theory explanation. Such use of alcohol and other drugs is a function of personal characteristics and factors related to the workplace and the culture of the work setting. In their study of young adult men and women, Mensch and Kandel (1988) found smoking among men significantly related to a number of job stressors, but only the dimension of work pressure was associated with alcohol use among men, and this relationship was weak. None of the other relationships between job stressors and drug use was significant for men, and no relationships were found for women. Certain limitations in the study may account for the lack of findings, mainly the use of indirect measures of job stressors and the narrow age distribution of the sample.

A certain amount of evidence has accumulated, however, suggesting that work-related stressors contribute to some degree to the extent of alcohol and other drug use. Tight deadlines and variance in work loads were found to relate to heavy, habitual drinking in a sample of Australian workers (Ferguson 1974). Higher work-role conflict emerged as a significant correlate of increased alcohol use among male and female managers (Havlovic and Keenan 1991). Role ambiguity, overload, and job insecurity have been shown to have a moderate, but significant, relationship to "escapist drinking" (Margolis et al. 1974), and employees are much more likely to consider a particular reason for drinking if they have experienced any one of eight work stressors (Fennell et al. 1981).

Seeman and Seeman (1992) demonstrated that chronic strains from ongoing work circumstances and intermittent life events plus high powerlessness typified a sample of men most vulnerable to high drinking quantity and problem drinking. The difference in drinking for those high versus low on these factors was highly significant. Finally, Watts and Short (1990) examined the relationship between job-related stressors and drug use among a mostly female sample of elementary and secondary school teachers. The correlations between the predictor variables and drug use were generally low. The strongest relationships occurred between job overload and alcohol use and between job stress and amphetamine, alcohol, and marijuana use.

In a large-scale study of men and women (Cohen et al. 1991), a combination of high job demands and low decision latitude for men was associated with increased probability of smoking. Women with greater marital conflict were significantly more likely to smoke and to drink moderate to heavy amounts of alcohol. Women in full-time employment had 110% greater odds of smoking, and if they also had high levels of marital conflict, they were more likely to drink at moderate to heavy levels. Marital conflict was associated with increased probability of smoking only among women not employed. The pattern of findings for women revealed a synergistic effect of marital conflict and work on drinking in contrast to an interaction of marital conflict and work in predicting smoking. These results underscore the importance of examining gender differences.

The research literature summarized indicates that work stressors do account for a certain amount of the variance in levels of psychiatric symptomatology and substance use and that the strength and consistency of these relationships appear to be greater between work stressor variables and indices of psychopathology than with substance use. This may be a function of a more direct relationship between stressors and psychopathology than is the case for substance use, which may be indirectly related to stressors through psychiatric distress.

One direction taken in recent research to build on knowledge derived from the study of job-related stressors has been to examine the contribution of both work and family stressors. Taking into account multiple risk factors across the domains of work and family is viewed as one way to generate models with potentially greater predictive power. However, the relationships that emerge when taking into account the combined aspects of work and family are not straightforward.

For example, occupying multiple roles does not necessarily place the individual at greater risk for negative health outcomes. In fact, there is evidence that being in multiple roles is associated with increased levels of well-being (Kandel et al. 1985) and that the accumulation of social roles is beneficial (Thoits 1983; Verbrugge 1983). Occupying multiple social roles may be especially important for women since they appear to have unique vulnerabilities in the role of spouse or partner. For example, women in general show higher levels of symptomatology than men in such areas as depression, and these differences are greatest among married persons (Cleary and Mechanic 1983). Interpersonal problems, especially marital conflict and dissatisfaction, are major stressors for women (Dytell et al. 1985).

Baruch et al. (1987) advanced the view that, for women, work may serve as a buffer against stressors encountered in other roles. They reported that the association between family role stress and negative health outcomes is most often found to be weaker in employed women as compared with homemakers. Similarly, Pearlin et al. (1981) found in a large-scale longitudinal study that women who occupied the role of homemaker were more likely to experience depression than employed women. Furthermore, Gove and Geerken (1977) reported that unemployed, married women reported more demands on them than did employed, married women but that both groups of women reported more demands on them than did married men. Homemakers also reported more symptoms of psychiatric symptomatology.

Even though involvement in work may serve as a buffer under certain conditions, the interplay of work and family roles is complex and may operate differently for men and women. For example, women in multiple roles reported lower family stress than work stress, yet family stress was more strongly related to negative mental health outcomes (Kandel et al. 1985). Similarly, Dytell et al. (1985) found that among women, family role stressors were more strongly related to psychological distress and physical illness variables than were work-related stressors. By contrast, among men, workplace stressors were more strongly related to symptoms of psychological distress, although family role stressors more strongly predicted actual physical illness.

In a community sample of married and unmarried individuals, with employed and unemployed in each group, Golding (1989) tested the hypothesis that, although role occupancy explains some variability in depression, perceptions of role-specific stress and support account for additional variability. Occupying both spouse and employee social roles was associated with low levels of depressive symptomatology. When marital and employment status were held constant, however, employment strain, supervisor support, and marital support in one role were associated with depression, regardless of occupancy of the other role. The author concluded that simultaneous consideration of role occupancy, stress, and social support facilitates the prediction of the conditions under which role occupancy will decrease depression.

Conflict between work and family roles is one set of conditions that clearly seems to affect the relationship between work-family stressors and psychiatric outcomes. Such conflict influences whether the accrual of new roles will exacerbate or buffer stresses experienced in other roles (Kandel et al. 1985). In addition to work stressors and family stressors, work-family conflict was highly correlated with depression among a sample of primarily female mental health employees (Carbone 1992). Also, blue-collar women who reported spillover between work and family in both directions had greater depression and anxiety than women who reported spillover in only one direction (Bromet et al. 1990). Moreover, the greater the perceived conflict between home and work roles, the more likely women were to report somatic complaints and depressed affect (Krause and Geyer-Pestello 1985). One potential factor contributing to women's experience of conflict is the pressure they feel to maintain high commitment in both work and family domains when they adopt the additional role of worker (Hall and Hall 1979), a factor that seems especially true for women with young children (Crouter 1984).

A number of other studies add further substantiation to the view that work and family role conflict is a risk factor of particular significance for women, although some findings suggest that it can increase risk for negative health consequences in men as well. In examining patterns of correlations among stressor, support, conflict, and satisfaction variables (Greenglass et al. 1988), greater interdependence between work and family spheres was found for women. On the other hand, more separation of work and family roles emerged for men. Conflict between job and family in women was related to higher incidence of depression, anxiety, and somatization. Similarly, in a study of Hispanic women professionals (Amaro et al. 1987), a combined gender and job model was most useful in explaining the findings in that both work and family factors (e.g., balancing demands of family and professional roles) were related to level of psychiatric symptomatology. This study also raises the question of how ethnicity interrelates as a risk factor for employees.

Another important employee characteristic is marital status. In examining the impact of multiple demands of job and home responsibilities on male and female single parents, Burden (1986) found single female parents to be at substantial risk for high levels of job and family role strain and decreased physical and emotional well-being. The potential vulnerability of men, as well as women, was shown in a study reported by Frone et al. (1991). In this case, the influences of work stressors, family stressors, and work-family conflict each made an independent contribution for both men and women to the prediction of psychological distress, even after controlling for the influence of a number of sociodemographic and psychosocial variables.

Finally, three studies provide support for the relationship between work-family role conflict and alcohol use. Parker and Harford (1992) analyzed data on men and women from a national longitudinal survey and found interactions of job pressure and gender-role attitudes related to increased alcohol consumption. Greater alcohol consumption was found with employed traditional women and egalitarian men who believe they have substantial obligations at home and who have high job competition. In addition, women with job pressures and substantial obligations at home experience a burden that can lead to greater alcohol use (Ehrensaft 1980). Likewise, a combination of full-time employment and high level of marital conflict was related to an increased likelihood of moderate to heavy drinking among women (Cohen et al. 1991). These studies indicate that the pressures of role expectations at home combined with high job demands may produce a psychological conflict that acts as a risk factor for those vulnerable to drinking behavior.

In summary, studies concerning the relationship between work and family stressors and psychiatric symptomatology provide empirical evidence in support of proposed stress models that posit direct and indirect relationships between key risk factors and negative health outcomes. A variety of job stressors ranging from work load to role conflict and ambiguity to organizational role stress are associated with higher levels of symptom-atology across gender, occupation, and role status subgroups. The relationship between job stressors and substance use also has been substantiated to some degree, although the patterns of these relationships are less clear. Intervening variables appear to play a major, although not well-understood, role in how job-related risk factors influence substance use behavior. Finally, family stressors, especially those associated with marital and parenting roles, appear at first glance to affect the level of symptomatology more among women than men. However, a closer examination of the data reveals a more complex pattern and suggests that the interrelationships between demands of employment and family need to be examined in the contexts of gender and family life phase to determine more clearly what conditions lead to similar or different outcomes for men and women.

PROTECTIVE FACTORS OF SOCIAL SUPPORT AND COPING: RELATIONSHIP TO PSYCHIATRIC OUTCOMES

A stress model is not complete unless consideration is given to the role of protective, as well as risk, processes. Although risk factors increase the likelihood of negative psychiatric outcomes, the potentially adverse influences of these factors can be mitigated if certain protective factors are available to the individual and are effectively utilized. Two protective factors of significance in this regard are social support and coping strategies. Each of these has received considerable attention in research on work and family stress.

Social support in one's environment can have a direct relationship to psychiatric outcomes, or it can buffer the harmful influences of risk factors. The likelihood of observing a direct effect will depend on whether one assesses the degree to which an individual is integrated into a large social network. Alternatively, a buffering effect is more likely to emerge if one assesses the perceived availability of interpersonal resources responsive to the needs elicited by stressful situations (Cohen and Wills 1985). Both types of effects have been observed in this area of stress research. How well either of these processes occurs will depend not only on the availability of support and the responsiveness of network members but on the individual's efforts to build and utilize supportive resources.

Individuals with supportive relations generally do better on a number of adjustment indices than those without such ties (Ganellen and Blaney 1984; Ganster et al. 1986). Social support is associated with low levels of depression (Aneshensel 1986; Billings and Moos 1982b; Schaefer et al. 1981), and reduced levels of social support have been related to various indices of psychological distress and psychiatric symptomatology (Eaton 1978; Hirsch 1979; Lin et al. 1979).

A number of research investigations have differentiated nonwork and work sources of support to examine their impact on individual adjustment. Nonwork sources of support include those from spouse, family, and friends. In this domain, marital support has been shown consistently to be associated with lower levels of depressive symptomatology (Caplan et al. 1976; Golding 1989; Vanfossen 1981). Brown and Harris (1978) found that women with confiding, intimate relations had one-fourth the incidence of depression as those with high stress and little support. Gutierres and Saenz (1992) found that for men, health problems increased with high stress but were moderated by social support from family. In contrast, although women's health problems also increased under conditions of high stress, they were not moderated by social support from family. In longitudinal studies, social support was found to predict improvements in mental health (Williams et al. 1981), to be associated with lower levels of depression (Aneshensel and Frerichs 1982), and to be related to psychological well-being (Turner 1981).

Work sources of support include supervisors and coworkers. Social support from supervisors or coworkers has been associated, directly or indirectly, with decreased anxiety (Himle et al. 1989) and decreased depression (Himle et al. 1989; Holahan and Moos 1982; LaRocco et al. 1980), lower levels of psychophysiologic symptoms (Schonfeld 1990), decreased incidence of burnout (Constable and Russell 1986; Dignam and West 1988; Eisenstat et al. 1981; Himle et al. 1989; Pines 1983; Ross et al. 1989), and lower work stress and strain (Haines et al. 1991;

Jayaratne et al. 1988; Shankar and Famuyiwa 1991).

A similar pattern of findings has emerged from a series of studies examining various combinations of nonwork and work sources of support and their effects on employee adjustment. LaRocco et al. (1980) conducted a meta-analysis including a variety of occupations and concluded that social support may mitigate the relationship of perceived job stress and strain for the general mental health of employees. Hendrix et al. (1988) found that job support was negatively correlated with burnout for men and women—a finding consistent with that reported by Cronin-Stubbs and Rooks (1985)—but that life support was negatively correlated with burnout for men only. Finally, social support from work and nonwork sources was negatively related to somatic complaints and depression (Fusilier et al. 1987), and, in a study of male doctors, those who reported higher social support (both in number and satisfaction) perceived less stress and reported lower anxiety and better general well-being (Kumari and Sharma 1990).

The second protective factor of interest is coping. A range of coping strategies is possible in responding to the demands of stressful conditions—some adaptive and some maladaptive. Coping is a process involving cognitive and behavioral efforts to manage the demands on one's resources (Lazarus 1991). As in the case of social support, the extent to which an individual learns and applies a range of effective coping strategies will influence how well this process provides a protective function.

Coping strategies that appear to serve as protective factors involve active behavioral and cognitive approaches as opposed to emotion-focused or avoidance strategies. Long and Gessaroli (1989) reported that problem-solving coping was inversely related to work stressors in a sample of teachers, and Srivastava and Singh (1988) found that approach coping markedly alleviated the negative effects of role stress on mental health. Pearlin et al. (1981) observed an indirect relationship between positive appraisal and depression. Positive appraisal modified economic strain and subjective feelings of mastery of the situation, which in turn affected depressed mood. Other studies provide further substantiation for the moderating effect of problem-focused coping on stressors (Bhagat et al. 1991; Shinn et al. 1989) and for the positive relationship between problem-focused coping and adjustment (Aldwin and Revenson 1987; Felton and Revenson 1984). In contrast, evidence is quite consistent that emotion-focused coping is associated with poor mental health outcomes (Kuehlmann 1990; Shinn et al. 1989) and that the causal relationship between emotion-focused coping and poor adjustment may be bidirectional (Aldwin and Revenson 1987; Felton and Revenson 1984).

Some evidence suggests that gender influences the style of coping utilized and the extent to which coping is effective in reducing negative outcomes. Folkman and Lazarus (1980) found that men used problem-focused coping longer than women, but the difference was possibly more attributable to sources of stress than to styles of coping within similar contexts. Women did have more health-related episodes associated with emotion-focused coping. Defares et al. (1984) reported that men employed more active and cognitive-based coping styles, whereas women used social support mechanisms in dealing with problems at work. The comparative effectiveness of social support and coping is somewhat unclear. In a study of working parents (Shinn et al. 1989), social support was a less powerful predictor of outcomes than individual coping. However, in an earlier study (Shinn et al. 1984), a larger effect was found for social support than for individual coping in reducing distress at work. Billings and Moos (1981) reported that coping is more important than social resources for men but equally important for women.

Research concerning the effects of avoidance coping (e.g., choosing to ignore the situation) quite uniformly indicates that this style of coping is related to poorer adjustment and increased use of substances. Snow and Kline (1991b) found that avoidance coping was highly related to greater psychological symptomatology and increased use of alcohol and tobacco. These findings are consistent with other research in which avoidance coping is positively related to higher levels on stressor variables (Long and Gessaroli 1989) and intensifies the negative effects of role stress on mental health (Srivastava and Singh 1988). The consistent pattern of findings regarding avoidance coping strongly suggests that it be included as a risk, rather than protective, factor in stress research.

Studies of social support and coping as protective factors provide further evidence for the usefulness of applying a stress, social support, and coping paradigm to work and family stress research. Both types of protective processes have been shown to have direct, positive effects on adjustment or to serve as moderators of the stressor-symptomatology relationship, depending on the nature of the variables under investigation. Although some coping strategies are clearly related to positive outcomes, others such as emotion-focused and avoidance coping are quite consistently linked to poorer adjustment and are better considered as risk factors. Gender differences in the utilization of social support and in the types of coping strategies employed may account for certain differences in outcomes observed for men and women. Finally, an important area for further study involves examining the interrelationship between social support and coping to understand their separate and combined contributions to psychiatric outcomes.

EFFECTIVENESS OF WORKPLACE INTERVENTIONS

Guided by theoretical models of the stress process, research evidence has accumulated, as indicated, linking certain risk and protective factors to psychiatric outcomes. Although current knowledge about these complex relationships is incomplete, the findings do provide an initial basis for designing and evaluating workplace interventions. In the area of research on work and family stress, these interventions involve the selection and application of various methods aimed at reducing specified work and family stressors as risk factors or enhancing social support and coping in work and nonwork domains as protective factors, or both.

Three major categories of intervention programs are delineated in the literature: quality of work life, health promotion, and employee assistance (Sonnenstuhl 1988). The first two of these categories can be classified as preventive interventions since they focus on either deterring the onset of psychiatric problems in the general population or improving employee mental health and reducing substance use among those at risk of developing more serious disorders.

Quality of work life programs are conceptualized from a systems perspective and therefore involve efforts to change organizational conditions or processes. The goals of such programs are to reduce or remove stressors at their source in the workplace, change the individual's role in the setting, or both. Examples of strategies used are job redesign or cooperative decision making. The importance of intervening at the organizational level is widely recognized because of the potential for broad-based impact (Ganster et al. 1982; Heaney and van Ryn 1990). From this perspective, efforts to enhance individual resilience are viewed as less effective if stressful conditions in the workplace remain unaltered. Implementation of system-level interventions requires sanction from the organization and participation from personnel at multiple hierarchical levels in the workplace. However, because it can be difficult to obtain necessary managerial support for these types of interventions, systems approaches aimed at effecting changes in employee well-being are less likely to be selected than are individual-centered types of interventions. Three studies that did target organizational stressors utilized various intervention methods—increased employee social support and work-team functioning (Heaney et al. 1992), increased employee participation (Jackson 1983), and work redesign (Wall and Clegg 1981)—and demonstrated reductions in reported psychiatric symptomatology.

Health promotion programs represent the broadest category of individual-focused preventive interventions. Theoretical underpinnings drawn from social learning theory (e.g., Bandura 1977) and stress and coping models (e.g., Lazarus and Folkman 1984; Pearlin and Schooler 1978) inform the design of interventions to promote individuals' self-efficacy and adaptive skills. These approaches are conceptualized primarily under the rubric of coping-skills training. Programs typically include any one or combinations of the following four levels of skill development: 1) enhancing problem solving, interpersonal communication, assertiveness, and related skills to improve employees' ability to reduce stressors at their source; 2) teaching cognitive appraisal processes that help control the meaning of stressful experiences;

3) promoting the effective utilization of social resources; and 4) training in stress management approaches such as biofeedback, progressive muscle relaxation, mental imagery, and other specific cognitive-behavioral techniques. This latter skill area refers to methods that help to manage stress after it has emerged.

Several comprehensive reviews of the literature on health promotion and stress management have been reported. Authors of the earliest compilation concluded that program evaluations were rare and that the evaluations that had been conducted were derived more often from professional opinions than from formal tests of effectiveness (Newman and Beehr 1979). Subsequent reviews indicated that methodological problems evident in many of the studies conducted in the 1970s and early 1980s raised concerns about the validity of reported findings (McLeroy et al. 1984; Murphy 1984). A meta-analysis of stress management programs conducted by Nicholson et al. (1988) showed "mildly encouraging results," but many programs were eliminated due to design limitations. Only 18 of 62 published reports could be analyzed in common. The need for rigorous studies of intervention effectiveness employing more adequate controls was clearly indicated. Ivancevich et al. (1990) highlighted selected coping-skills intervention studies that employed more rigorous methodology through the use of control groups, multiple outcomes, and longitudinal quasi-experimental or experimental designs. Despite improvements in workplace intervention research over the last 10 years, the reviewers reiterated that many evaluations of intervention programs continue to be hindered by methodological limitations such as inadequate control groups, difficulty in obtaining a sizable and randomized sample, and other threats to internal and external validity.

Only a limited number of coping-skills intervention studies employ relatively rigorous experimental or quasi-experimental designs and include psychiatric indicators as outcome variables. However, these studies do provide some initial evidence for intervention effectiveness in reducing psychiatric problems, such as depression, anxiety, somatic complaints, and substance use.

Positive results of coping-skills interventions have been reported for men and women from various occupational groups. For example, a stress reduction program conducted by the army led to lower levels of depression, anxiety, and hostility in a treatment group as compared with a control group (Harig et al. 1992). When a sample consisting of predominantly of female employees was taught to recognize and reappraise their interpretations of stressful events at work as less stressful, they reported a significant but modest decrease in depression and anxiety (Ganster et al. 1982). In a group of studies that involved three different occupational populations—supervisors (predominantly male), nurses, and teachers—coping-skills training led to fewer reported psychological symptoms, including somatic complaints (Raymer et al. 1992). Efforts to improve the coping skills of individual male and female employees and their work groups, simultaneously, resulted in reduced depression and somatization among a group designated as at risk for leaving their jobs. The individuals also reported positive changes in self-perceptions of their ability to handle stress at work (Heaney et al. 1992).

In a multicomponent intervention, women on public assistance were taught to identify stressors in their lives, to learn problem-solving techniques, and to practice problem redefinition and interpersonal coping skills (Tableman et al. 1982). The program participants improved more than control subjects on measures of depression, anxiety, and inadequacy. The authors emphasized that the positive outcomes were due to the inclusion of a variety of coping skills in their program rather than any single method. They also underscored the need to offer behavioral training rather than purely cognitive methods such as rethinking the problem or stress reappraisal.

Several studies have utilized multiple comparison groups to assess the effectiveness of coping-skills interventions. Two studies using mental health outcome variables included both male and female employees. Sallis et al. (1987) compared three conditions in which one group was offered a relaxation-training program; a second group participated in an intervention that combined relaxation, cognitive, and behavioral (i.e., assertiveness) techniques; and a third condition was designed as an educational support group. The study employed a longitudinal pretest, posttest, and 3-month follow-up design. All three groups were equally effective at reducing psychiatric symptoms (e.g., depression, anxiety, hostility). The comparability of findings suggests that the effectiveness of these programs may be attributable to nonspecific factors or that any skill improvements are beneficial if it is also assumed that even the support group members gained skills through their teaching of one another. Interestingly, the interventions were less effective at reducing perceived work stress. This finding supports Heaney and van Ryn's (1990) contention that coping-skills programs may be more likely to affect general indices of adjustment than specific work-related indices.

A second study (Goodspeed and DeLucia 1990), in which the majority of participants were women, involved two approaches to enhancing coping skills. A comparison of the two approaches again yielded comparable results, even over time. The Time-Life program involved the selection and practice of new coping strategies, whereas use of the Meyers-Briggs instrument involved identifying natural personality proclivities and goal setting to capitalize on personal strengths. Both groups had significant reductions in strain operationalized as somatic, behavioral, and cognitive symptoms. However, a high attrition rate with no analysis of its effect weakens this study's findings.

In contrast to the two previously described studies, Cecil and Forman (1990) attempted to affect stress and coping variables and found that not all types of intervention programs produce comparable results. In their study, three groups of teachers were divided into stress inoculation training (relaxation and cognitive restructuring), coworker support (listening and problem solving), and control (assessment only) groups. Only the stress inoculation training group reported reduced stress and enhanced coping skills.

Finally, there also are examples of successful multicomponent coping-skills programs sponsored by corporations as an ongoing aspect of their health promotion efforts. Three studies evaluating the effects of such programs have observed reductions in depression, anxiety, and hostility (Collings 1984); anxiety and somatic symptoms (Manuso 1980); and alcohol use (Wilbur et al. 1986).

Overall, the studies reviewed indicate that coping-skills interventions can have beneficial effects on psychiatric symptomatology. Research has not yet differentiated which program components are most effective in producing change and for whom. Although progress clearly has been made in the field of workplace intervention research aimed at reducing stress-related disorders, investigations that are guided by theoretical models, that pay attention to gender and other sample characteristics, and that clearly explicate the intervention content and format remain priorities for future research.

EXAMPLE OF WORKPLACE PREVENTIVE INTERVENTION: THE YALE WORK AND FAMILY STRESS PROJECT

The Yale Work and Family Stress Project involves studies in two major areas: 1) the evaluation of the effectiveness of work-based coping-skills interventions in reducing negative psychological and behavioral consequences of work and family stressors, and 2) the examination of the relationships between selected risk and protective factors and psychological symptomatology, substance use, and work adjustment indices. The conceptual framework for these investigations is a stress, social support, and coping paradigm (e.g., Lazarus and Folkman 1984) in which we assume there is a directional relationship between critical risk and protective factors and multiple psychological and behavioral outcomes. Within this model, work and family stressors and maladaptive coping strategies, such as avoidance coping, serve as risk factors. On the other hand, perceived social support and the use of more adaptive coping strategies operate as protective factors.

For purposes of the present chapter, we report on a study that involves an evaluation of the immediate and longer term effectiveness of a 15-session, workplace, coping-skills intervention for female employees. The intervention was designed to teach participants new strategies for reducing the negative influence of identified risk factors and for enhancing the beneficial effects of protective factors. We hypothesized that women who received the intervention, as compared with no-treatment control subjects, would report: 1) lower levels of employee role, work-family, and work environment stressors; 2) higher perceived social support from work and nonwork sources; 3) lower avoidance and higher behavioral and cognitive coping; 4) lower psychological symptomatology; and 5) lower tobacco, alcohol, and illicit drug use.

We expected these results to emerge at the immediate posttest and to remain evident at the 6-month follow-up. By the 22-month follow-up, we expected the initial effects to have attenuated.

Method

Participants.   Participants were 239 female, clerical workers employed at one of four job sites in Connecticut-based corporations. Site 1 was a large manufacturing company; sites 2, 3, and 4 were components of utility and telecommunications companies. Of the original sample, 136 employees participated in the intervention, and 103 served as control subjects. The overall sample was predominantly white (83%), had completed high school or vocational training (43%) or some college (46%), had worked in the company for an average of 9.4 years, and had an annual family income ranging from less than $30,000 (37%) to more than $50,000 (36%). Participants' mean age was 40.2 years, with about half (53%) of the women having children living at home.

The posttest sample consisted of 205 employees, representing 85.8% of the original sample. Of this number, 125 employees had participated in the intervention, and 80 were control subjects. The sample at 6-month follow-up consisted of 185 employees (77.4% of the original sample). Of these employees, 110 were intervention participants, and 75 were control subjects. At the 22-month follow-up, 158 employees (66.1% of the original sample) remained in the panel. Of these, 90 employees were intervention participants, and 68 were control subjects. The proportions of intervention and control participants across each of the demographic categories remained relatively constant across all three time periods.

Procedures.   Participants were recruited first by circulating a program description to all eligible employees within each workplace inviting their participation. It was explained that half of those who volunteered would be randomly selected to receive the intervention and half would serve as control subjects. This procedure was followed to protect against bias resulting from volunteer effects. It also was explained that all participants would complete a set of research measures prior to and at the completion of the intervention (4 months later), and at 6- and 22-month follow-up periods. Next, employees were randomly assigned within each site to the program or control conditions. Those selected for the intervention met in small groups of approximately 10–12 employees led by a facilitator for 1.5 hours each week for a 15-week period. Sessions were held at the company site and occurred during work hours, with each company providing release time to support employee participation.

Intervention. The intervention was based on a tripartite conceptual model of coping and adaptive behavior: attacking the problem, rethinking the problem, and managing the stress. The model is derived from Pearlin and Schooler's (1978) hierarchy of coping mechanisms: 1) responses that change the situation, 2) responses that control the meaning of the stressful experience, and 3) responses that function to control the stress after it has emerged and when it cannot be removed at the source.

The first component of the intervention focused on methods that potentially could limit the source of the stress by using proactive techniques that eliminate or reduce the need for ongoing stress management. The second component concentrated on techniques that do not eliminate the stressor but that help to modify the cognitive appraisal processes that lead to or exacerbate the perception of stress. Cognitive restructuring and other methods that change how the problem is assessed and understood were central to this component. The third component focused on teaching specific stress management techniques. Strategies included progressive relaxation and mental imagery exercises, which participants were taught to engage in by themselves outside of the training to ensure skill acquisition. The final portion of the intervention was used to integrate concepts and techniques introduced in previous sessions and to facilitate each participant's development of a personal stress management plan. Throughout the training, participants were encouraged to develop a range of adaptive behaviors and to substitute them for maladaptive tension-reduction behaviors such as substance use. A more detailed outline of the intervention sessions is provided in Table 8–1.

Table 8–1. Coping with work and family stress: outline of intervention sessions

Session I: Women, multiple roles, and stress

Participants identify diverse roles they assume and the kinds of pressures they face while satisfying the demands of each role. Role conflict is examined as a particularly difficult problem. The causes, symptoms, and possible consequences of stress faced by working women are examined.

Session II: Identifying and examining stressful situations

Participants identify problem situations from their own experiences. They learn to analyze problems as the first step in mastering them by utilizing their own individual resources as well as those of a supportive group.

Session III: Problem solving

Procedures for rational problem solving are learned and practiced. As a group, participants generate various problem-solving strategies and consider the costs and benefits of those strategies.

Session IV: Managing the stress (part A)

Deep breathing and muscle relaxation are utilized as means for ameliorating the physical and psychological impact of stress. Ongoing practice of these techniques continues throughout the program so that participants will become reasonably expert with them.

Session V: Attacking the problem (part A)

The benefits and elements of effective communication and assertiveness are discussed. Participants practice these communication skills in work- and family-related situations.

Session VI: Attacking the problem (part B)

Empathic listening and responding are employed as communication skills.

Session VII: Attacking the problem (part C)

Participants express their needs directly, effectively, and assertively and learn to identify and overcome barriers to effective communication.

Session VIII: Attacking the problem (part D)

All the communication skills are brought together and practiced as means for changing conditions that may cause difficulties and stress for the individual.

Table 8–1.	Coping with work and family stress: outline of intervention sessions *(continued)*

Session IX: Personal networks and social support

Participants consider "significant others" and members of their social networks as sources of support in time of need. Enhancement of the personal network and the costs and benefits of social support are discussed.

Session X: Group strategies

Some problems can best be addressed by a group of people acting together. The group mobilization process is considered as an option with its own strengths and weaknesses.

Session XI: Rethinking the problem (part A)

Often, the way one thinks about a situation influences the severity of the stress experienced. Effective and ineffective styles for assessing the impact of a stressor and various kinds of statements people make to themselves in these situations are identified and practiced.

Session XII: Rethinking the problem (part B)

The participants share the ways in which they have thought through recent personal situations and the consequences of those thoughts for stress and self-esteem. Alternative ways of thinking about these situations are considered.

Session XIII: Managing the stress (part B)

Participants develop their imaginations through visualization exercises and self-suggestion as ways to reduce the effects of stress.

Session XIV: Personal stress management plan (part A)

Problem-solving, cognitive restructuring, and stress management techniques are integrated as each participant considers the costs and benefits of applying each strategy to situations drawn from family and work experiences. A systematic procedure for sorting through these options is introduced.

Session XV: Personal stress management plan (part B)

Participants will continue to develop the personal stress management plan. Implementation of this plan in gradual steps is discussed. Participants will also review their accomplishments during the program and process termination issues.

Measures. Participants completed the Work and Family Stress Questionnaire, a self-report instrument that included sections on demographic information; family history of health problems; and assessments of risk and protective factors, psychological adjustment, and substance use. The measure for demographic characteristics elicited information concerning participants' age, race, marital status, education, length of employment, family income, and number and ages of children living at home. Family history of health problems was assessed by asking participants to indicate the presence or absence of major diseases among their primary blood relatives.

Three of the risk factors assessed were work and family stressors. A measure of employee role stress was obtained using the Role Quality Scale (Baruch and Barnett 1986). Respondents indicated to what extent each of the items is currently a source of concern or demand for them. Internal consistency for this scale was quite high (Cronbach's α = .90). Work-family stress was derived from items on the questionnaire developed specifically for this project (Cronbach's α = .81). These items assess the extent to which demands from employment and family are perceived as too extensive, conflictual, or overlapping. Work environment stress (Cronbach's α = .59) was determined by asking participants whether selected environmental conditions in their immediate work location (e.g., noise, temperature, health hazards) were perceived as stressors. The fourth risk factor assessed was avoidance coping, obtained from the Health and Daily Living Form (Billings and Moos 1982a), which assesses individuals' strategies for addressing problem situations or events. Those items on the avoidance subscale that pertained to substance use were eliminated due to their direct relationship to the dependent measures. The correlation between this modified scale and the original avoidance scale was very high (Pearson's r = .93).

Two of the protective factors consisted of work and nonwork sources of social support. These factors were assessed using an adaptation of House's (1980) measure of perceived social support. Participants rated the extent to which their supervisor, coworkers, spouse/partner, family, and friends were perceived as supportive regarding difficulties both at home and at work. Ratings pertaining to supervisor and coworkers were combined to create a measure of social support from work sources (Cron-bach's α = .88), and those for spouse/partner, family, and friends were combined to create a measure of social support from non-work sources (Cronbach's α = .90). The other protective factors included behavioral and cognitive coping, the two other sub-scales obtained from the Health and Daily Living Form.

Three measures of psychological symptomatology were em-ployed. The state-anxiety subscale of the Spielberger State-Trait Anxiety Inventory (Spielberger et al. 1970) was used as a measure of transitory feelings of tension, apprehension, and heightened autonomic nervous system activity. Participants were asked to rate whether or not they were currently experiencing 20 anxiety-related mood states. Spielberger et al. found the reliability coeffi-cients (Cronbach's α) for this subscale to range from .83 to .92. The Center for Epidemiologic Studies—Depression (CES-D) Scale was utilized to assess current level of depressive symptom-atology and depressive affect. Participants rated 20 items, indi-cating the frequency of their occurrence during the last week. The CES-D has been found to have high internal consistency, with reliability coefficients (Cronbach's α) ranging from .85 to .90. The CES-D also has proven useful in discriminating between samples of psychiatric patients and the general population (Radloff 1977). The Cohen-Hoberman Inventory of Physical Symptoms (Cohen and Hoberman 1983) is carefully designed to include many phys-ical symptoms that have been viewed traditionally as psychoso-matic while excluding symptoms of an obvious psychological nature. Participants were asked to indicate how much each of 39 common physical symptoms had bothered or distressed them during the past 2 weeks. This inventory has been found (Cohen and Hoberman 1983) to have adequate internal consistency (Cronbach's α = .89).

Current substance use was assessed using a self-report format adapted from the National Survey on Drug Abuse (Miller et al. 1982). Participants were asked to indicate both the frequency and amount of usage in the past 30 days of the following substances: cigarettes, caffeine, alcohol, marijuana or hashish, sedatives, tran-quilizers, stimulants, pain killers, cocaine or crack, and LSD. Although there are some questions regarding the validity of self-report measures of substance use, studies support both the reliability and validity of these measures (Akers et al. 1983; Johnston et al. 1984). In addition, participants were asked to rate the extent to which they tried to reduce tension by drinking more, smoking more, or taking more tranquilizing drugs.

The final set of dependent variables was obtained through a factor analysis that included all psychological symptomatology scales and substance use items described. A principal-component factor analysis with varimax rotation was used; factors with eigenvalues ≥ 1 were retained. Items loading together on a factor were evaluated for internal consistency using Cronbach's alpha. Items with item-scale correlations < .40 were dropped. Variables were created by standardizing retained items using z scores and combining them with equal weighting. The analysis yielded four factors: 1) psychological symptomatology (anxiety, depression, and somatic complaints), 2) alcohol use, 3) illicit drug (marijuana, cocaine, and crack) use, and 4) tobacco use.

Results

A high level of participation in the intervention was attained. The mean ± SD number of sessions completed by participants was 11.9 ± 3.4, with 85.2% of the intervention group completing 10 or more sessions. Univariate analyses of covariance were conducted to compare intervention and control groups at posttest and at 6- and 22-month follow-ups on each of the risk and protective factors and dependent variables were adjusted for pretest scores. Regarding the outcome variables, in addition to assessing program impact on psychological symptomatology, the three scales of this measure also were analyzed separately to determine whether there were any differential effects of the intervention on anxiety, depression, and somatic complaints over time. Even though these scales loaded on the psychological symptomatology factor, they also have a certain degree of independence from each other (correlations ranged from .54 to .66) and are meaningful dimensions of psychological adjustment to assess in their own right. Finally, due to the very limited reporting of illicit drug use, the results for this variable are of questionable validity and are not included in the following summary of results.

Intervention effectiveness at posttest.   Intervention participants reported (see Table 8–2) significantly lower employee role
stress ($F = 4.88$; df = 1,202; $P < .05$), higher social support from
work sources ($F = 5.52$; df = 1,202; $P < .05$), lower psychological
symptomatology ($F = 6.99$; df = 1,200; $P < .01$), fewer depressive
symptoms ($F = 4.97$; df = 1,200; $P < .05$), fewer somatic complaints ($F = 6.82$; df = 1,200; $P < .01$), and less tobacco use ($F =
6.84$; df = 1,176; $P < .01$). They also tended to report greater use of
behavioral coping strategies ($F = 2.74$; df = 1,184; $P < .10$) and less
anxiety ($F = 2.92$; df = 1,201; $P < .10$).

Intervention effectiveness at 6-month follow-up.   At 6-month
follow-up (see Table 8–3), intervention participants reported a
lower level of work environment stress ($F = 5.38$; df = 1,182; $P <$

Table 8–2.   Least squares means ± standard errors and F ratios on
stressor, social support, coping, and outcome variables at
posttest

Variable	Intervention	Control	F	df
Stressor				
Employee role	−.086 ± .062	.134 ± .077	4.88[*]	1,202
Work/family	−.043 ± .069	.067 ± .086	.99	1,202
Work environment	.011 ± .079	−.017 ± .099	.05	1,202
Social support				
Nonwork sources	.031 ± .065	−.048 ± .081	.58	1,202
Work sources	.092 ± .062	−.143 ± .078	5.52[*]	1,202
Coping				
Behavioral	19.18 ± .592	17.56 ± .774	2.74[†]	1,184
Cognitive	17.27 ± .536	16.83 ± .701	.24	1,184
Avoidance	2.46 ± .191	2.74 ± .248	.83	1,183
Outcomes				
Psychological symptoms	−.269 ± .173	.467 ± .217	6.99[**]	1,200
Anxiety	−.075 ± .076	.132 ± .094	2.92[†]	1,201
Depression	−.099 ± .074	.164 ± .092	4.97[*]	1,200
Somatic complaints	−.100 ± .064	.169 ± .080	6.82[**]	1,200
Tobacco use	−.172 ± .113	.313 ± .146	6.84[**]	1,176
Alcohol use	−.142 ± .139	.218 ± .180	2.52	1,176

[*]$P < .05$; [**]$P < .01$; [†]$P < .10$

.05), higher social support from work sources ($F = 5.45$; df = 1,182; $P < .05$), lower avoidance coping ($F = 9.62$; df = 1,159; $P < .01$), lower psychological symptomatology ($F = 9.49$; df = 1,175; $P < .01$), less anxiety ($F = 14.29$; df = 1,178; $P < .001$), fewer somatic complaints ($F = 5.03$; df = 1,177; $P < .05$), and less alcohol use ($F = 5.42$; df = 1,154; $P < .05$). They also tended to report greater use of behavioral coping strategies ($F = 2.77$; df = 1,159; $P < .10$) and fewer depressive symptoms ($F = 3.41$; df = 1,175; $P < .10$).

Intervention effectiveness at 22-month follow-up. The only significant program effect observed at the 22-month follow-up (see Table 8–4) was that intervention participants continued to

Table 8–3. Least squares means ± standard errors and F ratios on stressor, social support, coping, and outcome variables at 6-month follow-up

Variable	Intervention	Control	F	df
Stressor				
Employee role	−.062 ± .078	.067 ± .094	1.09	1,182
Work/family	−.081 ± .082	.120 ± .099	2.45	1,182
Work environment	−.124 ± .084	.182 ± .102	5.38[*]	1,182
Social support				
Nonwork sources	−.005 ± .078	-.000 ± .095	.00	1,182
Work sources	.128 ± .082	-.175 ± .100	5.45[*]	1,182
Coping				
Behavioral	18.60 ± .644	16.85 ± .830	2.77[†]	1,159
Cognitive	16.72 ± .596	16.32 ± .767	.17	1,159
Avoidance	2.17 ± .192	3.15 ± .247	9.62[**]	1,159
Outcomes				
Psychological symptoms	−.365 ± .197	.597 ± .242	9.49[**]	1,175
Anxiety	−.182 ± .076	.271 ± .093	14.29[***]	1,178
Depression	−.092 ± .084	.154 ± .103	3.41[†]	1,175
Somatic complaints	−.090 ± .073	.167 ± .089	5.03[*]	1,177
Tobacco use	−.148 ± .135	.185 ± .173	2.30	1,155
Alcohol use	−.267 ± .199	.491 ± .257	5.42[*]	1,154

[*]$P < .05$. [**]$P < .01$; [***]$P < .001$; [†]$P < .10$

report fewer somatic complaints ($F = 4.17$; df = 1,149; $P < .05$). However, a number of other differences reached a trend level of significance. Program participants also reported higher social support from nonwork sources ($F = 3.54$; df = 1,155; $P < .10$), greater use of behavioral ($F = 3.35$; df = 1,130; $P < .10$) and cognitive ($F = 3.07$; df = 1,133; $P < .10$) coping strategies, and less use of tobacco ($F = 3.67$; df = 1,123; $P < .10$) and alcohol ($F = 2.76$; df = 1,128; $P < .10$).

Attrition analyses. The attrition rate was 14.6% at posttest, 22.6% at 6-month follow-up, and 33.9% at 22-month follow-up. A significantly higher rate of attrition occurred in the control group

Table 8–4. Least squares means ± standard errors and F ratios on stressor, social support, coping, and outcome variables at 22-month follow-up

Variable	Intervention	Control	F	df
Stressor				
Employee role	−.011 ± .081	−.029 ± .093	.02	1,155
Work/family	.050 ± .095	−.056 ± .109	.54	1,155
Work environment	−.077 ± .092	.112 ± .106	1.79	1,155
Social support				
Nonwork sources	.120 ± .087	−.132 ± .100	3.54[†]	1,155
Work sources	.060 ± .086	−.068 ± .099	.95	1,155
Coping				
Behavioral	18.76 ± .740	16.68 ± .868	3.35[†]	1,130
Cognitive	17.96 ± .634	16.24 ± .747	3.07[†]	1,133
Avoidance	2.77 ± .261	2.88 ± .310	.08	1,132
Outcomes				
Psychological symptoms	-.096 ± .217	.154 ± .257	.55	1,141
Anxiety	.018 ± .091	−.008 ± .104	.04	1,153
Depression	−.010 ± .099	.038 ± .114	.10	1,144
Somatic complaints	−.104 ± .081	.153 ± .096	4.17[*]	1,149
Tobacco use	−.191 ± .164	.289 ± .190	3.67[†]	1,123
Alcohol use	−.168 ± .220	.397 ± .258	2.76[†]	1,128

[*]$P < .05$; [†]$P < .10$

(22.3%) than in the intervention condition (8.8%) at posttest ($\chi^2 =$ 8.55, df = 1, $P < .003$), but this difference did not occur at subsequent follow-ups. To assess potential threats to external validity, chi-square analyses were conducted comparing stayers and dropouts at posttest and at both follow-ups on the demographic variables, and multivariate analyses of variance (MANOVAs) were completed comparing the two groups at the three time periods on mean pretest levels for the stressor, social support, coping, and dependent variables. To test for potential threats to internal validity, MANOVAs were conducted to assess condition by attrition status interactions utilizing pretest scores on the study variables. Given potential threats to the validity of study findings posed by attrition, a significance level of .10 was chosen for the attrition analyses to reduce the likelihood of Type II error (i.e., the failure to detect true differences when they occur) (Snow et al. 1992; Tebes et al. 1992).

None of these analyses was significant at posttest. At the 6-month follow-up, no differences were observed between stayers and dropouts on demographic variables, and only two differences were found on the pretest levels of the other study variables. Dropouts reported a higher level of work-family stress ($F =$ 3.42; df = 1,235; $P < .07$) and lower social support from work sources ($F = 9.20$; df = 1,235; $P < .01$) at pretest than stayers. No condition-by-attrition status interactions were significant. At the 22-month follow-up, a somewhat different pattern of attrition findings emerged. Single employees were more likely to drop out than either married or separated/divorced employees ($\chi^2 = 5.28$, df = 2, $P < .08$), and dropouts reported higher levels of employee role stress ($F = 3.21$; df = 1,235; $P < .08$) and tobacco use ($F = 2.69$; df = 1,216; $P < .10$) at pretest than stayers. In addition, three condition-by-attrition status interactions were significant. Program dropouts reported higher levels of support from nonwork sources at pretest than program stayers, whereas there were no differences between control stayers and dropouts ($F = 2.84$; df = 1,235; $P < .10$). An opposite effect occurred for social support from work sources. Program dropouts reported lower levels of support as compared with program stayers, whereas the differences were again negligible between control stayers and dropouts ($F = 4.27$; df = 1,235; $P < .05$). Finally, program dropouts reported higher alcohol use at pretest than program stayers, whereas control dropouts reported lower pretest alcohol use than control stayers ($F = 4.85$; df = 1,216; $P < .05$).

Discussion

This research examined the effectiveness of a coping-skills intervention within a longitudinal study design. The study was guided by a paradigm in which key risk and protective factors are assumed to have a directional relationship to psychological and behavioral outcomes. Based on this paradigm, the intervention was designed to effect changes in selected stressor, social support, and coping variables. It was expected that changes in these variables would be accompanied by reductions in psychological symptomatology and substance use over time.

At posttest and at the 6-month follow-up, variables in each of the identified domains were positively affected by the intervention. Among the risk factors, the intervention had an immediate positive effect on employee role stress. Six months later, program participants indicated lower work environment stress and less use of avoidance coping than did control subjects. No differences, however, were observed between the groups on the work-family stressor variable. Among identified protective factors, intervention participants reported higher perceived support from work sources and, to some degree, greater use of behavioral coping strategies. Changes in these risk and protective factors were paralleled by reductions in psychological and substance use outcomes. Participants reported lower psychological symptomatology at both time periods. Based on the scales making up this factor, the intervention had a significant positive effect on depressive symptoms at posttest, a highly significant impact on anxiety by 6-month follow-up, and a consistently positive effect on somatic complaints at both time periods. In addition, participants reported lower tobacco use at posttest and lower alcohol use at the 6-month follow-up. This pattern of findings is consistent with that reported by Sallis et al. (1987), suggesting that it is more difficult to induce change in work-related stressors than in general indexes of adjustment.

The overall results from the present study indicate that interventions focusing on coping-skills enhancement offered within the workplace can be of substantial benefit to working women in secretarial and clerical positions. Moreover, the findings complement those observed in related studies with other subgroups of women (Ganster et al. 1982; Raymer et al. 1992; Tableman et al. 1982), supporting broader generalizability of the effectiveness of coping-skills interventions for women.

Another goal of this research was to examine the longer term effectiveness of the intervention. Analyses revealed that the extent and magnitude of program effects observed at earlier time periods had attenuated by 22-month follow-up. The intervention had no continuing impact on risk factors. Three longer term effects were found for protective factors but only at a marginal level of significance. Program participants tended to report higher social support from nonwork sources and greater use of both behavioral and cognitive coping strategies. It appears that the intervention may have positive spillover into nonwork domains later in time and that the intervention's focus on increasing the range and quality of coping strategies contributed to the longer term effects for these protective factors. It is reasonable to assume that a person-centered, coping-skills intervention has more potential to change individual behavior than to decrease risk factors linked to organizational conditions. Regarding the outcome variables, the significant positive effect of the intervention on somatic complaints was still maintained by 22-month follow-up. Clearly, the intervention had a consistent impact over time on the number and extent of physical symptoms reported by program participants. Lower tobacco use also was reported by program participants; however, as compared with the finding at immediate posttest, this difference was now only marginal. Finally, the positive program effect for alcohol use at 6-month follow-up remained at a trend level of significance 22 months after the intervention, although the validity of this latter finding is questionable.

The attrition findings support the external validity of the observed results, with only limited restrictions in the generalizability of study findings occurring at the 6- and 22-month follow-up periods. The analyses also lend support to the internal validity of the results at the posttest and 6-month follow-up, since no condition-by-attrition status interactions were significant at either time period. Two significant condition-by-attrition status interactions at the 22-month follow-up suggest that the positive effect observed for social support from nonwork sources was most likely even stronger, whereas the positive alcohol effect was likely spurious.

Several patterns from the results are noteworthy. One pattern indicates that the intervention can have a positive impact on modifying risk and protective factors, at least up to 6 months after the intervention. Immediate and shorter term effects applied mostly to work-related domains such as employee role and work environment stressors and support from work sources. This may be due to the setting of the intervention. The opportunity to learn skills and share experiences with colleagues in small groups at the workplace may have contributed to increases in social support from work sources, particularly from coworkers, and to reductions in perceived work-related stressors. Strategies, such as the involvement of other family members and a greater concentration on the overlap between work and family demands, may be necessary to achieve more significant change in family-related risk and protective factors and in the level of work-family conflict.

A second pattern is the appearance of sleeper, or delayed, effects. For example, although differences between program and control groups on protective factors (social support from work sources and use of behavioral coping) remained constant from posttest to 6-month follow-up, the lower use of avoidance-coping strategies and alcohol by program participants, and the much stronger effect in reducing levels of reported anxiety, did not emerge until the follow-up period. These variables were linked conceptually in the intervention curriculum where alcohol use was examined as an avoidant response to stress and work-family conflicts and as a means often used to reduce tension or anxiety. The parallel decrease in these three areas at follow-up suggests that this approach to reducing participants' substance use was effective. These findings underscore the need for longitudinal assessment of workplace interventions to capture program effects that require additional time to emerge as participants are able to apply new skills necessary to produce behavioral change.

Finally, the relative lack of findings at the 22-month follow-up raises questions about what influences the maintenance of effects over longer time periods. Some investigators are now testing the efficacy of "booster" sessions to reinforce initial positive effects. The lack of long-term results also may be, in part, a methodological issue. Longitudinal research, especially in natural settings such as workplaces, is often adversely affected by panel loss due to a variety of nonprogram factors. The rate of attrition in this study, especially by 22-month follow-up, may have resulted in insufficient power to detect positive program effects in a number of areas. Comparison of group means suggests that both attenuation of real effects and reduction of power may be operating. It is also possible that changes in the work environments over the 2 years counteracted positive program influences (e.g., increased stressful work conditions, less supportive work environment). During the 2 years following the intervention, the companies all experienced severe transitions due to a more difficult economic climate.

CONCLUSION

The development of effective workplace preventive interventions depends on the integration of risk and protective factor research with intervention research. Models of the stress process guide research on risk and protective factors and their relationships with specified outcomes and, in turn, are modified on the basis of empirical findings. These same models provide frameworks for designing interventions aimed at modifying factors that, according to theory or empirical evidence, will most likely lead to positive outcomes. Ideally, evaluation of interventions should occur within the context of risk and protective factor assessments with the same study sample to validate whether the salient factors identified in such analyses are those targeted and affected by the intervention (Snow and Kline 1991a).

In this chapter, we reviewed research on work and family risk and protective factors and their relationships to psychiatric outcomes as well as research on the effectiveness of workplace interventions in reducing psychiatric symptomatology. A number of important conceptual issues and research problems are apparent from this review that need to be addressed to make further advances in this area of stress research.

First, regarding risk and protective factor research, the relationships among these factors and psychiatric outcomes are complex and require more specific delineation regarding the situational contexts and processes that affect the nature and pattern of relationships. As a result, current models need to account better for whether hypothesized relationships among variables remain constant across domains (e.g., work and family), situational contexts (e.g., occupational role and status or stage of family development), and sociodemographic subgroups (e.g., gender or marital status), and, if they vary, what explains the different patterns that are observed. Another issue of relevance is whether selected risk and protective factors operate differently in relation to specific psychiatric outcomes (e.g., the positive relationship found between coworker support and marijuana use on the job among women [Mensch and Kandel 1988] as compared with the common finding of negative relationships between social support indices and psychiatric symptomatology). A question that follows is whether unique subsets of factors, and therefore different models, better explain one type of psychiatric outcome than another (e.g., depression and anxiety versus substance use). Also, models should attempt to explain on what basis bidirectional, as opposed to unidirectional, relationships would be assumed to operate (e.g., how role strain can be both a cause and a consequence of psychiatric disorder [Link et al. 1990]) in order to generate transactional models of the stress process. Finally, models of the stress process need to address under what conditions direct versus moderating or mediating effects of coping and social support would be expected to emerge.

Issues pertaining to intervention research also need to be addressed. Given the multifaceted nature of coping-skills and stress management programs, there is a need to delineate the specific contribution of each of the intervention components to changes in outcome variables (Snow and Kline 1991a). One approach to this problem would be to utilize additional control groups to isolate training-specific effects of various skill enhancement or stress management strategies (Murphy 1986). Further, since coping skills are central components of workplace interventions, comparisons need to be made to determine whether using a variety of coping strategies is more effective in reducing stressors and stress-related problems than use of only one type of strategy (Pearlin and Schooler 1978). If so, this area of investigation also would involve testing the effectiveness of combinations of coping strategies. Finally, it cannot be assumed that a given intervention has the same degree of effectiveness for all participants. Evaluation of the differential effectiveness of coping-skills interventions across various high-risk subgroups (e.g., single-parent mothers, lower income individuals), in conjunction with the intervention component analyses discussed, would provide further specification of the best type of intervention in a given situation.

The second set of research issues centers on problems of measurement. The lack of clear support for the construct validity of stressor measures is a problem of central importance in this area of research. Investigators often rely on measures of stressful conditions and measures of distress that are very similar operationally, raising the possibility that they are assessing a single concept (Brief and Atieh 1987). Items on scales designed to measure the level of a stressor variable often identify stressful conditions by distressing effects (Schonfeld 1990). Meier (1991) reported that measures of stress, depression, and anxiety are typically highly intercorrelated and that such findings weaken claims of discriminant validity for occupational stress measures. A related problem is the reliance on a single method measurement approach, typically self-reports. The use of multimethod assessment approaches by supplementing self-reports with physiological and other objective measures would improve research designs and would allow comparisons of objective and perceptual measures of conditions within the workplace and family. Another problem in this area of research is how to assess the extent to which stressors in one particular domain (e.g., work) are related to reported levels of psychiatric symptomatology. Frone et al. (1991) asserted that this relationship may be overestimated if the concurrent influences of stressors from other domains as well as individual differences in psychosocial resources and vulnerabilities are not controlled.

Matters related to research design also require further attention. To determine more definitively whether the positive effects
on psychiatric outcomes observed in certain coping-skills intervention studies are the result of participants' skill acquisition,
placebo or attention control conditions need to be incorporated
into study designs. Although such alternative conditions would
include certain elements comparable to the experimental condition (e.g., release time for employees, meeting in small groups),
they would not include specific coping-skills training. Use of
these types of controls would help rule out alternative explanations that observed differences are due to generalized or other
nonspecific program effects rather than to the coping-skills training per se. Another critical issue is that workplace preventive
interventions remain, for the most part, person-centered. Although these are valid and meaningful approaches, one criticism
is that they rely on teaching individuals how to adapt to stressful
conditions rather than undertaking efforts to change system-
level conditions within the workplace or family more directly
(Heaney and van Ryn 1990). Until constraints on this type of
research can be better addressed, the impact of system-level
change efforts, or combinations of system-level and person-
centered designs, on psychiatric outcomes remains essentially
untested. Finally, much of the research in the area of work and
family stress has relied on cross-sectional designs, leaving many
questions regarding cause-and-effect relationships. Longitudinal
risk and protective factor research is needed to examine the interrelationships of these variables with psychiatric symptomatology
over time. Causal modeling, and other statistical methods, then
could be applied to test alternative "best-fit" models to explain
the relationship among variables across various time periods.
Similarly, the use of longitudinal designs in workplace intervention research would allow testing the maintenance of program
effects, whether delayed or sleeper effects emerge over time, and
whether the inclusion of repeated interventions at selected time
intervals increases program impact.

Research in the area of work and family stressors and their
relationships to psychiatric consequences has progressed substantially over the past decade. Further advances will depend on
refinement in the explanatory models used to guide this work, on

resolution of problems inherent in existing research methodology, and on utilization of more comprehensive and sophisticated research designs.

REFERENCES

Akers RL, Massey J, Clarke W, et al: Are self-reports of adolescent deviance valid? biochemical measures, randomized response, and the bogus pipeline in smoking behavior. Social Forces 62:234–251, 1983

Aldwin CM, Revenson TA: Does coping help? a reexamination of the relation between coping and mental health. J Pers Soc Psychol 53:337–348, 1987

Amaro H, Russo NF, Johnson J: Family and work predictors of psychological well-being among Hispanic women professionals. Psychology of Women Quarterly 11:505–521, 1987

Aneshensel CS: Marital and employment role-strain, social support, and depression among adult women, in Stress, Social Support, and Women. Edited by Hobfoll SE. New York, Hemisphere, 1986, pp 99–114

Aneshensel CS, Frerichs RR: Stress, support, and depression: a longitudinal causal model. Journal of Community Psychology 10:363–376, 1982

Aro S, Hasan J: Occupational class, psychosocial stress and morbidity. Annals of Clinical Research 19:62–68, 1987

Bandura A: Social Learning Theory. Englewood Cliffs, NJ, Prentice-Hall, 1977

Baruch GK, Barnett RC: Role quality, multiple role involvement, and psychological well-being in midlife women. J Pers Soc Psychol 51:578–585, 1986

Baruch GK, Biener L, Barnett R: Women and gender in research on work and family stress. Am Psychol 42:130–136, 1987

Bhagat RS, Allie SA, Ford DL Jr: Organizational stress, personal life stress and symptoms of life strains: an inquiry into the moderating role of styles of coping. Journal of Social Behavior and Personality 6:163–184, 1991

Billings AG, Moos RH: The role of coping responses and social resources in attenuating the impact of stressful life events. J Behav Med 4:139–157, 1981

Billings AG, Moos RH: Stressful life events and symptoms: a longitudinal model. Health Psychol 1:99–118, 1982a

Billings AG, Moos RH: Work stress and the stress buffering roles of work and family resources. Journal of Occupational Behavior 3:215–232, 1982b

Boxer PA, Wild D: Psychological distress and alcohol use in fire fighters. Paper presented at the American Psychological Association and National Institute for Occupational Safety and Health Conference, Washington, DC, November 1992

Brief AP, Atieh JM: Studying job stress: are we making mountains out of molehills? Journal of Occupational Behavior 8:115–126, 1987

Bromet EJ, Dew MA, Parkinson DK, et al: Predictive effects of occupational and marital stress on the mental health of a male workforce. Journal of Organizational Behavior 9:1–13, 1988

Bromet EJ, Dew MA, Parkinson DK: Spillover between work and family: a study of blue-collar working wives, in Stress Between Work and Family. Edited by Eckenrode J, Gore S. New York, Plenum, 1990, pp 133–151

Brown GW, Harris T: Social Origins of Depression: A Study of Psychiatric Disorder in Women. London, Tavistock, 1978

Burden DS: Single parents and the work setting: the impact of multiple job and homelife responsibilities. Family Relations 35:37–43, 1986

Caplan RD, Robinson EAR, French JRP Jr, et al: Adhering to Medical Regimens: Pilot Experiments in Patient Education and Social Support. Ann Arbor, MI, Institute for Social Research, 1976

Carbone DJ: Correlates of depression in mental health employees. Paper presented at the American Psychological Association and National Institute for Occupational Safety and Health Conference, Washington, DC, November 1992

Cecil MA, Forman SG: Effects of stress inoculation training and co-worker support groups on teachers' stress. Journal of School Psychology 28:105–118, 1990

Cleary, PD, Mechanic D: Sex differences in psychological distress among married people. J Health Soc Behav 24:111–121, 1983

Cohen S, Hoberman HM: Positive events and social supports as buffers of life change stress. Journal of Applied Social Psychology 13:99–125, 1983

Cohen S, Wills TA: Stress, social support, and the buffering hypothesis. Psychol Bull 98:310–357, 1985

Cohen S, Schwartz JE, Bromet EJ, et al: Mental health, stress, and poor health behaviors in two community samples. Prev Med 20:306–315, 1991

Collings CH: Stress and the workplace, in Behavioral Health: A Handbook of Health Enhancement and Disease Prevention. Edited by Weiss SM, Hurd JA, Miller NE, et al. New York, Wiley, 1984, pp 1079–1086

Constable JF, Russell DW: The effect of social support and work environment upon burnout among nurses. Journal of Human Stress 2:20–26, 1986

Cooper CL, Baglioni AJ Jr: A structural model approach toward the development of a theory of the link between stress and mental health. Br J Med Psychol 61:87–102, 1988

Cronin-Stubbs D, Rooks CA: The stress, social support, and burnout of critical care nurses: the results of research. Heart Lung 14:31–39, 1985

Crouter AC: Spillover from family to work: the neglected side of the work-family interface. Human Relations 37:425–442, 1984

Defares PB, Brandjes M, Nass CH, et al: Coping styles and vulnerability of women at work in residential settings. Ergonomics 27:527–545, 1984

Dignam JT, West SG: Social support in the workplace: tests of 6 theoretical models. Am J Community Psychol 16:701–724, 1988

Donat DC, Neal B, Addleton R: Situational sources of stress for direct care staff in a public psychiatric hospital. Psychosocial Rehabilitation Journal 14:76–81, 1991

Dytell RS, Pardine P, Napoli A: Importance of occupational and non-occupational stress among professional men and women. Paper presented at the meeting of the Eastern Psychological Association, Philadelphia, PA, March 1985

Eaton WW: Life events, social supports, and psychiatric symptoms: a reanalysis of the New Haven data. J Health Soc Behav 19:230–234, 1978

Ehrensaft D: When women and men mother. Sociology Review 49:37–73, 1980

Eisenstat RA, Felner RD, Kennedy M, et al: Job involvement and the quality of care in human service settings. Paper presented at the annual meeting of the American Psychological Association, Los Angeles, CA, August 1981

Felton BJ, Revenson TA: Coping with chronic illness: a study of illness controllability and the influence of coping strategies on psychological adjustment. J Consult Clin Psychol 52:343–353, 1984

Fennell ML, Rodin MS, Kantor GK: Problems in the work setting, drinking, and reasons for drinking. Social Forces 60:114–132, 1981

Ferguson D: A study of occupational stress and health, in Man Under Stress. Edited by Welford AT. New York, Wiley, 1974, pp 83–98

Folkman S, Lazarus RS: An analysis of coping in a middle-aged community sample. J Health Soc Behav 21:219–239, 1980

French JRP, Caplan RD: Organizational stress and individual strain, in The Failure of Success. Edited by Marrow AJ. New York, Amacon, 1973, pp 30–66

Frone MR, Russell M, Cooper ML: Relationship of work and family stressors to psychological distress: the independent moderating influence of social support, mastery, active coping, and self-focused attention. Journal of Social Behavior and Personality 6:227–250, 1991

Fusilier MR, Ganster DC, Mayes BT: Effects of social support, role stress, and locus of control on health. Journal of Management 13:517–528, 1987

Ganellen RJ, Blaney PH: Hardiness and social support as moderators of the effects of life stress. J Pers Soc Psychol 47:156–163, 1984

Ganster DC, Mayes BT, Sime WE, et al: Managing organizational stress: a field experiment. J Appl Psychol 67:533–542, 1982

Ganster DC, Fusilier MR, Mayes BT: Role of social support in the experience of stress at work. J Appl Psychol 71:102–110, 1986

Golding JM: Role occupancy and role-specific stress and social support as predictors of depression. Basic and Applied Social Psychology 10:173–195, 1989

Goodspeed RB, DeLucia AG: Stress reduction at the worksite: an evaluation of two methods. American Journal of Health Promotion 4:333–337, 1990

Gove WR, Geerken MR: The effect of children and employment on the mental health of married men and women. Social Focus 56:66–76, 1977

Greenglass ER, Pantony K-L, Burke RJ: A gender-role perspective on role conflict, work stress and social support. Journal of Social Behavior and Personality 3:317–328, 1988

Gutierres SE, Saenz D: Occupational stress and health among Anglo and ethnic minority university employees. Paper presented at the American Psychological Association and National Institute for Occupational Safety and Health Conference, Washington, DC, November 1992

Haines VA, Hurlbert JS, Simmer C: Occupational stress, social support and the buffer hypothesis. Work and Occupations 18:212–235, 1991

Hall FS, Hall DT: The Two Career Couple. Reading, MA, Addison-Wesley, 1979

Harig PT, Price VA, Oleshansky M, et al: U.S. Army War College stress management programs: type-A behavior reduction. Paper presented at the American Psychological Association and National Institute for Occupational Safety and Health Conference, Washington, DC, November 1992

Harris MM, Fennell ML: A multivariate model of job stress and alcohol consumption. Sociology Quarterly 29:391–406, 1988

Havlovic SJ, Keenan JP: Coping with work stress: the influence of individual differences. Journal of Social Behavior and Personality 6:199–212, 1991

Heaney CA, van Ryn M: Broadening the scope of worksite stress programs: a guiding framework. American Journal of Health Promotion 4:413–420, 1990

Heaney CA, Price RH, Rafferty J: A preventive intervention to increase employee coping resources: enhancing work relationships and improving work team functioning. Paper presented at the American Psychological Association and National Institute for Occupational Safety and Health Conference, Washington, DC, November 1992

Hendrix WH, Cantrell RS, Steel RP: Effect of social support on the stress-burnout relationship. Journal of Business and Psychology 3:67–73, 1988

Himle DP, Jayaratne S, Thyness P: The effects of emotional support on burnout, work stress and mental health among Norwegian and American social workers. Journal of Social Service Research 13:27–45, 1989

Hirsch BJ: Psychological dimensions of social networks: a multimethod analysis. Am J Community Psychol 7:263–277, 1979

Holahan CJ, Moos RH: Social support and adjustment: predictive benefits of social climate indices. Am J Community Psychol 10:403–415, 1982

Hollinger RC: Working under the influence (WUI): correlates of employees' use of alcohol and other drugs. Journal of Applied Behavioral Science 24:439–454, 1988

House JS: Occupational Stress and the Mental and Physical Health of Factory Workers. Ann Arbor, MI, Institute for Social Research, 1980

House JS, McMichael AJ, Wells JA, et al: Occupational stress and health among factory workers. J Health Soc Behav 20:139–160, 1979

House JS, Victor S, Helen L, et al: Occupational stress and health among men and women in the Tecumseh community health study. J Health Soc Behav 27:62–77, 1986

Ivancevich JM, Matteson MT: Stress and Work. Glenville, IL, Scott, Foresman, 1980

Ivancevich JM, Matteson MT, Freedman SM, et al: Worksite stress management interventions. Am Psychol 45:252–261, 1990

Jackson SE: Participation in decision making as a strategy for reducing job-related strain. J Appl Psychol 68:3–19, 1983

Jayaratne S, Himle D, Chess WA: Dealing with work stress and strain: is the perception of support more important than its use? Journal of Applied Behavioral Science 24:191–202, 1988

Johnston LD, O'Malley PM, Bachman JG: Drugs and American High School Students 1975–1983. Rockville, MD, National Institute on Drug Abuse, 1984

Kahn RL, Byosiere A: Stress in organizations, in Handbook of Industrial and Organizational Psychology. Edited by Dunnette M. Chicago, IL, Rand-McNally, 1990, pp 571–650

Kahn RL, Wolfe DM: Organizational Stress: Studies in Role Conflict and Ambiguity. New York, Wiley, 1964

Kandel DB, Davies M, Raveis VH: The stressfulness of daily social roles for women: marital, occupational, and household roles. J Health Soc Behav 26:64–78, 1985

Karasek R, Gardell B, Lindell J: Work and non-work correlates of illness and behavior in male and female Swedish white collar workers. Journal of Occupational Behaviour 8:187–207, 1987

Krause N, Geyer-Pestello HF: Depressive symptoms among women employed outside the home. Am J Community Psychol 13:49–67, 1985

Kuehlmann TM: Coping with occupational stress among urban bus and tram drivers. Journal of Occupational Psychology 63:89–96, 1990

Kumari K, Sharma S: Social support, organizational role stress and well-being: a study of medicos. Psychological Studies 35:163–169, 1990

Landsbergis PA: Occupational stress among health care workers: a test of the job demands-control model. Journal of Organizational Behavior 9:217–239, 1988

LaRocco JM, House JS, French JR Jr: Social support, occupational stress, and health. J Health Soc Behav 21:202–218, 1980

Lazarus RS: Psychological stress in the workplace. Journal of Social Behavior and Personality 6:1–13, 1991

Lazarus RS, Folkman S: Stress, Appraisal, and Coping. New York, Springer, 1984

Lin L, Simeone RS, Ensel WM, et al: Social support, stressful life events, and illness: a model and an empirical test. J Health Soc Behav 20:108–119, 1979

Link BG, Mesagno FP, Lubner ME, et al: Problems in measuring role strains and social functioning in relation to psychological symptoms. J Health Soc Behav 31:354–369, 1990

Long BC, Gessaroli ME: The relationship between teacher stress and perceived coping effectiveness: gender and marital differences. Alberta Journal of Educational Research 35:308–324, 1989

Manuso J: Corporate mental health programs and policy, in Strategies for Public Health. Edited by Ng L, Davis D. New York, Van Nostrand Reinhold, 1980, pp 368–378

Margolis GL, Kroes WH, Quinn RP: Job stress: an unlisted occupational hazard. J Occup Med 16:659–661, 1974

McLeroy K, Green L, Mullen K, et al: Assessing the effects of health promotion in worksites: a view of stress program evaluations. Health Educ Q 11:379–401, 1984

Meier ST: Tests of the construct validity of occupational stress measures with college students: failure to support discriminant validity. Journal of Counseling Psychology 38:91–97, 1991

Mensch BS, Kandel DB: Do job conditions influence the use of drugs? J Health Soc Behav 29:169–184, 1988

Miller JD, Cisin IH, Gardner-Keaton H, et al: National survey of drug abuse: main findings 1982 (DHHS Publ No ADM-83-1263). Washington, DC, U.S. Government Printing Office, 1982

Moos RH, Swindle RW Jr: Stressful life circumstances: concepts and measures. Stress Medicine 6:171–178, 1990

Murphy LR: Occupational stress management: a review and appraisal. Journal of Occupational Psychology 57:1–15, 1984

Murphy LR: A review of organizational stress management research: methodological considerations. Journal of Occupational Behavior Management 8:215–228, 1986

Neale MS, Singer JA, Schwartz JL, et al: Yale-NIOSH occupational stress project. Paper presented at the 4th annual meeting of the Society of Behavioral Medicine, Baltimore, MD, March 1983

Newman JD, Beehr T: Personal and organizational strategies for handling job stress: a review of research and opinion. Personnel Psychology 32:1–43, 1979

Nicholson T, Duncan DF, Hawkins W, et al: Stress treatment: two aspirins, fluids, and one more workshop. Professional Psychology: Research and Practice 19:637–641, 1988

Oehler JM, Davidson MG, Starr LE, et al: Burnout, job stress, anxiety, and perceived social support in neonatal nurses. Heart Lung 20:500–505, 1991

Parker DA, Brody JA: Risk factors for alcoholism and alcohol problems among employed women and men, in Occupational Alcoholism: A Review of Research Issues (NIAAA Res Monogr No 8). Washington, DC, U.S. Government Printing Office, 1982, pp 99–128

Parker DA, Harford TC: Gender-role attitudes, job competition and alcohol consumption among women and men. Alcoholism: Clinical and Experimental Research 16:159–165, 1992

Pearlin LI, Schooler C: The structure of coping. J Health Soc Behav 19:2–21, 1978

Pearlin LI, Lieberman MA, Menaghan EG, et al: The stress process. J Health Soc Behav 22:337–356, 1981

Pines A: On burnout and the buffering effects of social support, in Stress and Burnout in the Human Service Professions. Edited by Farber BA. New York, Pergamon Press, 1983, pp 155–174

Price RH: The education of a prevention psychologist, in Preventive Psychology: Theory, Research and Practice. Edited by Felner RD, Jason LA, Moritsugu JN, et al. New York, Pergamon, 1983, pp 290–296

Radloff L: The CES-D scale: a self-report depression scale for research in the general population. Applied Psychosocial Measurement 1:385–401, 1977

Ratsoy EW, Sarros JC, Aidoo-Taylor N: Organizational stress and coping: a model and empirical check. Alberta Journal of Educational Research 32:270–285, 1986

Raymer KS, Sime WE, Setterlind S: The impact of occupational stress and interpersonal strain on the physical and emotional health of employees before and after. Paper presented at the American Psychological Association and National Institute for Occupational Safety and Health Conference, Washington, DC, November 1992

Ross RR, Altmaier EM, Russell DW: Job stress, social support, and burnout among counseling center staff. Journal of Counseling Psychology 36:464–470, 1989

Sallis JF, Trevorrow TR, Johnson CC, et al: Worksite stress management: a comparison of programs. Psychology and Health 1:237–255, 1987

Schaefer CJ, Coyne JC, Lazarus RS: The health-related functions of social support. J Behav Med 4:381–406, 1981

Schonfeld IS: Psychological stress in a sample of teachers. J Psychol 124:321–338, 1990

Seeman M, Seeman AZ: Life strains, alienation, and drinking behavior. Alcoholism: Clinical and Experimental Research 16:199–205, 1992

Shankar J, Famuyiwa OO: Stress among factory workers in a developing country. J Psychosom Res 35:163–171, 1991

Shinn M, Rosario M, Morch H, et al: Coping with job stress and burnout in the human services. J Pers Soc Psychol 46:864–876, 1984

Shinn M, Wong NW, Simko PA, et al: Promoting the well-being of working parents: coping, social support, and flexible job schedules. Am J Community Psychol 17:31–55, 1989

Snow DL, Kline ML: A worksite coping skills intervention: effects on women's psychological symptomatology and substance use. The Community Psychologist 24:14–17, 1991a

Snow DL, Kline ML: A worksite coping skills intervention with female employees: effects on psychological symptomatology and substance use. Paper presented at the Biennial Conference on Community Research and Action, Tempe, AZ, June 1991b

Snow DL, Tebes JK, Arthur MW: Panel attrition and external validity in adolescent substance use research. J Consult Clin Psychol 60:804–807, 1992

Sonnenstuhl WJ: Contrasting employee assistance, health promotion, and quality of work life programs and their effects on alcohol abuse and dependence. Journal of Applied Behavioral Science 24:347–363, 1988

Spielberger CD, Gorsuch RL, Lushene RE: State-Trait Anxiety Inventory Manual. Palo Alto, CA, Consulting Psychologists, 1970

Srivastava AK, Singh HS: Modifying effects of coping strategies on the relation of organizational role stress and mental health. Psychol Rep 62:1007–1009, 1988

Tableman B, Marciniak D, Johnson D, et al: Stress management training for women on public assistance. Am J Community Psychol 10:357–367, 1982

Tebes JK, Snow DL, Arthur MW: Panel attrition and external validity in the short-term follow-up study of adolescent substance use. Evaluation Review 16:151–170, 1992

Thoits PA: Multiple identities and psychological well-being: a reformulation and test of the social isolation hypotheses. American Sociological Review 48:174–187, 1983

Turner RJ: Social support as a contingency in psychological well-being. J Health Soc Behav 22:357–367, 1981

Vanfossen BE: Sex differences in the mental health effects of spouse support and equity. J Health Soc Behav 22:130–143, 1981

Verbrugge LM: Multiple roles and physical health of women and men. J Health Soc Behav 24:16–30, 1983

Wall TD, Clegg CW: A longitudinal study of group work redesign. Journal of Occupational Behavior 2:31–49, 1981

Watts DW, Short AP: Teacher drug use: a response to occupational stress. J Drug Educ 20:47–65, 1990

Wilbur CS, Hartwell TD, Piserchia PA: The Johnson & Johnson Live For Life program: its organization and evaluation plan, in Health and Industry. Edited by Cataldo MF, Coates TJ. New York, Wiley, 1986, pp 338–350

Williams AW, Ware JE Jr, Donald CA: A model of mental health, life events, and social supports applicable to general populations. J Health Soc Behav 22:324–336, 1981

Wilsnack RW, Wilsnack SC: Women, work, and alcohol: failures of simple theories. Alcoholism: Clinical and Experimental Research 16:172–179, 1992

Index

*Page numbers printed in **boldface** type refer to tables or figures.*

recovery phase of grief
and, 189
stress and increased risk of,
187

Transactional model
of life events and
psychological
disturbance, 23
of stress processes, 223
Traumatic events
assessment of, 142
bereavement and, 207
panic disorder and, 117–118
Treatment
of panic disorder and
posttraumatic stress
disorder, 142
of psychiatric
complications of
bereavement,
208–212
stress-reducing for
schizophrenia, 70–71
2-deoxyglucose (2DG), 76–82

Unipolar disorder. *See*
Depression

Vietnam War, combat stress
in veterans of, 149,
150–151, 153, 162, 165,
171–172
Violence, traumatic stressors
and panic disorder,
117–118
Vulnerability, to stressors
adverse reactions to minor
stressors, 31

and biological models of
mental illness, 16–17, 20
in bipolar patients, 96–98,
99–100
idiosyncratic appraisals
and depressive
reactions, 88–89

War neurosis, 153
Women. *See also* Gender
risk of psychiatric
complications of
bereavement in, 203
stress reactions to combat
exposure in, 158
study of affective disorders
and stress in, 100–106
work and family role
conflict as source of
stress, 229–231, 231–232
Workplace, stress in. *See also*
Occupation
development of effective
intervention
programs, 257
effectiveness of
interventions in,
237–257
models for study of,
221–225
relationship of to
psychiatric outcomes,
225–233
social networks and coping
strategies for, 233–237
World War II, combat stress
in veterans of, 153, 162

Yohimbe, 122